I]

IN THE CLASSROOM

PETER DANIEL MITSKINIS

PublishAmerica
Baltimore

First printing

PublishAmerica has allowed this work to remain exactly as the author intended, verbatim, without editorial input.

Softcover 9781462691630
PUBLISHED BY PUBLISHAMERICA, LLLP
www.publishamerica.com
Baltimore

Printed in the United States of America

I would like to dedicate my story to the following individuals who have always believed in me and have never doubted my dreams no matter how crazy they may have been. Without my close family and friends, this book could not have been completed.

Thank you,

Mom and Dad, my sister Stephanie, Grandma and Grandpa, Ivana Popowich, and Kate Ryan, for your love and family support.

John Spicer, Mary Ronan, Theodore Titus, Zita Van Oosten, and Anne Badali, for believing in my goals and dreams of becoming a teacher.

Natalie Lind, Tiffany Zigras, Paul Titanic and family, Terri (Theresa) Penney, and Jean Howard for your constant love, friendship and support!

A special dedication to my life-long friend Grace for your love, support and friendship.

MY JOURNEY

In order to live life to the fullest I believe that it is important for people to have positive attitudes towards life and others. To have a positive attitude the most important skill to acquire is interpersonal skills. Interpersonal skills have to do with the behaviours and feelings that exist within all of us, and influences the way we interact with others. Whether we are shy or bold, quiet or passive, domineering or cooperative, these are all examples of characteristics that relate to interpersonal skills. In order to be "good at life" it is important for us to get along with others. We live in a society where we rely on constant interaction with others; therefore, it is important that we learn to accept others for who they are and not judge individuals. I believe that it is imperative for all teachers to have strong interpersonal skills, because they deal with so many students, parents and other staff members each day, and they need to learn to feel comfortable with a variety of different people and personalities. I strive to be an educator who will enable students to become active participants in their educational journey. Teaching has always been a passion of mine, and I hope to work with individuals who have exceptionalities as well as students of all academic abilities. As an individual with a physical disability, I believe that I possess great gifts that allow me to connect to both students with and without disabilities.

Before I get into the reasons why I have chosen to pursue a career in the education field let me tell you a little bit about myself. I was born on June 9th, 1984. After nine months my mother was ready to give birth to her first born baby; a joyous occasion for many expectant mothers. After a long labour I finally arrived. However there were complications at birth; I was not breathing when I was born and was immediately rushed to Sick Kids Hospital in Toronto, Ontario where I called home for the next little while. As a result of my birth complications I am now living with cerebral palsy (CP). CP is a disability that affects an individual's movement or posture which is caused by brain damage. When I was born the umbilical cord was pinched during birth which prevents the flow of oxygen that is sent to the brain. This affects the delivery of messages being sent from the brain to tell different body parts how to function. There are many forms of CP, and depending on its severity this disability can affect individual's communication and mobility. My disability is neither progressive nor communicable. Although CP is not curable, individuals with CP can effectively live full lives with the appropriate education, therapy and technology.

The summer that I was born I spent a good part of it in the hospital. My parents, many family members and friends came to visit me to make sure I was doing well. About a month later, my parents were able to bring me home. My mom told me that I was a very fussy baby for the first couple of years. No one really knew that I had CP, until I was about 2-years-old. My parents had been connected with a therapist who told them that based on my physical characteristics there was a chance that I had CP. That year my parents brought me to a paediatrician and he was the person who told them right away that I did in fact have CP.

Growing up; I tried to become an active part of society despite my physical limitations. I attended regular Catholic schools where I was integrated into the regular classroom environment. I love school. It was a place where I could interact with my friends, learn new things, and develop meaningful relationships with people my own age.

Over the years my parents worked with me along with doctors, specialists, speech therapists and physiotherapists to seek ways to improve my walking and speech. I had a very hard time accepting my disability for many years, and still do now and then. I would not want to participate in activities with others who had disabilities, and no one in my circle of friends had a disability. It was difficult for me to come to grips with the fact that I had challenges and could not do the things that my friends were able to do. I had the mind of a physically able person, but a body of a physically challenged person. I wanted so much to be a part of the crowd, and participate on hockey teams, school sport teams, and simple activities such as riding public transit with my friends.

For the most part, my friends were very good with me and made me feel like I was a part of their groups. However, whenever we were on the school playground for recess, and they wanted to play games that I could not join, such as field hockey, tackle football, or even simple tag, this made me feel very upset and disconnected from my peers, as it was hard for me to participate. There were times when I would get so frustrated with my disability, and wished I could end my life right then and there. However, I had (and still have) a very supportive family and many caring friends who have helped me so much over the years to learn to accept myself for who I am. This story that I am about to share will explain the challenges that I have faced in my life, the obstacles that

I have overcome as well as the people who have helped me through it all.

CP is a very complex disability. There is no way in knowing how an individual will turn out when they are born with CP. CP is a disorder that affects individual's posture or movement and it is caused by brain damage. It affects the voluntary muscles which impairs ones communication and/or mobility. There are four main variations of CP, which are spastic, athetoid, ataxic, and mixed. In many cases you can't even tell if individuals even have CP.

I have spastic CP, which is the most common type to have. Nearly 80 per cent of individuals living with CP have this type. Some characteristics of my disability includes, one or more tight muscle groups, which limits my ability to move; stiff and jerky movements; and in some cases individuals have a hard time moving from one place to another. Although it is challenging to live with my disability, I am considered to be a very high functioning individual, which allows me to participate in many daily activities that others with more severe disabilities cannot.

When teachers have students with CP in their classroom it is important to create a supportive classroom environment that encourages these students to participate in every facet of the school day. Basic accommodations that I required as a student were extra time to complete assignments or tests, more time to get between classes, and a note taker or scribe to help me with writing in class. I have had the opportunity to work with students who also have CP over the years through my volunteer experiences in schools; however their cases were much more severe than mine. In these cases students need extra time to move around the school, they need to be corrected with their posture and fine motor skills, and it is important to encourage them to use assistive devices such as computers, to expedite their writing or even communication devices to help them interact with others.

Like many people with disabilities, it was important for my teachers to create a positive learning environment that was supportive to my physical needs and encouraged me to participate in every aspect of my learning experience. Although I was a very bright individual growing up, I required assistance to help me with everyday tasks that others do with such ease and take for granted. Through my elementary and secondary school years, I was provided with educational assistants and peer helpers who help guide and assist me with my daily classroom routines.

Research has shown that when schools implement inclusive education strategies in the general education classroom, this proves to be beneficial to all students. Inclusion of students with various exceptionalities is becoming more and more common in today's education system and has also become the "program of choice" for students with various disabilities, including those with intellectual disabilities, (Smith et al., 2006, 184). Full inclusion of students with exceptionalities received criticism in the early 1970s, and in the 1980s resource room programs were criticized. However, since the mid-1980s, there had been a call for a dual education system that includes students with exceptionalities in the regular classroom setting. Today Canadian publicly funded schools accept all students: those for whom English is a second language, aboriginal students, students with extraordinary gifts or talents, students with learning challenges such as autism or from the parental abuse of alcohol or drugs, prior to the student's birth and many more.

Students with exceptionalities who may have been segregated or denied education in the past, are now fully integrated in schools across the country with appropriate accommodations and modifications to meet their physical and academic needs. Inclusion can be very successful for many students; if the appropriate accommodations and modifications are put into place for them. It was very successful for me. The most common accommodation for students is providing them with an Educational Assistance (EA). EAs are employed by the School Boards to work one-on-one with students who require assistants beyond what the regular classroom teacher can provide.

MY EARLY YEARS

Growing up, I required an EA while I was in school to help me with daily classroom routines. I well never forget my very first EA; her name is Mrs. Anne Badali. Mrs. Badali is a kind and generous individual who is always willing to go out of her way for anyone, staff or student; family or friend. Students know her for her love, passion and dedication as an EA. Her outgoing and loving personalities are just some of the Christ-like qualities she possesses. I started kindergarten in 1989 at the age of five. This was my first year in a publicly funded school, and it was also Mrs. Badali's first time as an EA. EAs are hired by the school boards to help children and young adults with exceptionalities in the delivery of special education programs at all grade levels. Mrs. Badali did a fantastic job working with me. As we go through life, people walk in and out of our lives, but the ones that are important to us often leave a mark in our hearts. Like many important people in my life, Mrs. Badali helped mould me and shape me into the strong and energetic individual that I am today.

Starting school at the age of five can be a scary step for anyone to take. Although I do not remember my younger years that well, my parents have often told me how much I enjoyed kindergarten, and working with Mrs. Badali. I had the privilege of having her a second time around when I was in grade 4. Over the years I have kept in touch with her and we have shared our life stories together. She has always told me of how proud she is of my accomplishments, and how she will never forget me since I was her very first student as an EA. I remember after I had finished grade 4 Mrs. Badali was reassigned to a new school where she began working at the high school around the corner, where I eventually ended up going. I will never forget how upset I was when she left. She was a great assistant and she is still a wonderful friend. She was like a third parent to me in my early years, and she always made me feel so good about myself. Fortunately I do keep in touch with Mrs. Badali and see her from time to time. Whenever I volunteer at St. Brother Andre Catholic High School, where I was once a student, and where Mrs. Badali is presently an EA, I see her working with students, and I notice how happy they are to be in her company.

EAs are amazing individuals who take the time to work with children who have exceptionalities. Their job is very demanding and stressful at times. It is important for teachers and administrators to constantly recognize their efforts and once in a while thank them for all that they do for students. It can be challenging for parents to accept their son or daughters exceptionality, and sending them to school can be a scary thing for them. It is important for parents to get to know their child's EA and special education teacher, to see what they do with their child and the services that are provided to them.

The job of an EA can be very hectic at times. Through my volunteer experiences in special education departments within the York Catholic School Board, I have had the privilege of meeting a number of wonderful EAs. For most part the EAs that I have met enjoy working with children who have exceptionalities. The true genuine EA is so easy to point out. This individual is kind towards students and staff members; always willing to help those who are in need of their assistance;

respects other teachers and those in administrative positions, and is passionately a people person. If I were in charge of hiring EAs, these are the qualities that I would look for in a candidate. I would like to thank Ms. Anne Badali for being the amazing person she is, and for continuing to bring smiles to other students with exceptionalities.

* * *

When parents find out their son or daughter has CP, there is no way in telling them what the future holds for their child. However, it is important to get them fully involved in society as much as possible. My parents did an excellent job in providing me with a high quality life style. We would spend summers at our cottage, which I did not fully enjoy because having a disability made it challenging to get around the Canadian Rock. However, I really enjoyed our many trips down south to Florida where my grandparents have a house and now my parents have a place of their own as well. I also participated in a number of after-school activities that helped me with my walking. I was involved in horse back riding to help improve my posture, indoor swimming lessons, where the pool was 90 degrees, which helped relax my muscles, as well as down hill skiing, physiotherapy, and indoor soccer. All of these activities have helped me develop my muscles and improved my ability to walk independently. Many times I would fight and resist my parents and physiotherapists; I was often frustrated whenever I did my exercises. However, looking back I am glad that they managed to do as much as they did with me, because today I am capable of doing so much more for myself.

As an individual with CP I am considered to be very high functioning. Many doctors and specialists had a hard time offering ways to improve my walking, because I was doing so well. I started walking independently at the age of 6, with a little help. The following year I was planning on receiving my First Holy Communion in the Catholic Church. This is a significant milestone for young Catholics; as we believe that the Communion is the actual body and blood of our Lord and Saviour Jesus Christ. That year it was my goal to walk down the Church aisle without using my walker. I remember that day so well. My family and close friends were all present to watch me receive my First Holy Communion. That year I had so much support from my teachers, therapists, parents and grandparents. My parents really encouraged me to work hard and practice my walking. I remember my parents telling me that the more I worked on my walking and exercises, the better I would get.

My parents are amazing people who have done so much for my sister and I. They have helped us in so many ways and have loved us both unconditionally. As a teacher, my dad would spend hours with me in elementary school, helping me with homework and projects. His guidance and creative teaching strategies helped me get through my elementary school days with ease. My mom did everything she could to help me succeed as well. When I was young she gave up her career in advertising and stayed home to watch my sister and me. To earn extra money for food, trips, nice clothes, she ran her own daycare program from home. Although there were times when I did not enjoy coming home to crying babies and children taking their afternoon naps in my room, I now understand the importance of family, and how much my mom sacrificed her career to be there for her children.

Everyday I would come home from school where I would find a warm snack, which was usually some kind of baked good or leftovers from the night before. I love to eat and still do. You would never know to see me, I'm a pretty slender guy, but I enjoy a good hardy meal. My mom is a great cook, and always takes pride in her meals. I am so proud of my mom, she is now working for a marketing company, where she has a very good job and is often able to work from home.

Dinner at my house has always been a family tradition. The four of us always sat around the kitchen table and for many years my grandparents, mom's parents, lived with us, and when they were home, they joined us too. As Catholics the six of us always begin a meal with a prayer. We thanked God each night for the food we were about to receive and for one another. My grandmother was the one who taught me how to pray as a kid, and each night we would also pray together before bed. I loved having my grandparents live with us. Although they were in Florida a good portion of the year, it was always comforting to have extra adults around the house growing up, whenever they were in town.

While attending grade-school I grew up in a middle class neighbourhood in Markham, Ontario. It was a quaint town where everybody knew my name. As a little boy I loved life. I was always cheerful and everyone loved my smile. I had tons of friends and was known as "Mr. Popularity." It was important for me to do well in school and achieve all that I could. Over the years I probably changed my mind on what profession I wanted to pursue hundreds of times. I remember always telling people that I wanted to be a Chartered Accountant just like my late Uncle Jimmy. "Why?" People would ask me. I just knew that I wanted to be "a somebody" back then, and usually people valued you based on your wealth. My uncle was a wealthy man, and I wanted the same lifestyle as he did. My favourite subject in school was math. I enjoyed it very much and did well in it. My parents were so pleased with how well I was doing both academically and physically. I was the kind of student who always worked hard to achieve good marks.

My uncle Jimmy was actually one of my dad's first cousins. Growing up I always admired him. He had a wonderful wife, Krista, and two beautiful children. For years I wanted to be just like my uncle; rich, a family man, and fun to be around. I always wanted him to be a part of my life.

* * *

I was very popular in elementary school. Everyone knew me for my wonderful personality, million dollar smile, and of course my clothes. Many teachers always said that my sister and I were the best dressed kids in the school. I remember each year before school began; my family would take a family trip to Rochester, New York where we visited my dad's cousins. It was on these trips that my mom and cousins would take my sister and I back-to-school shopping. My mom found great pleasure in dressing her children. She always bought us quality clothes that would last me many years. I probably still have a few clothing items from my high school days as I am not that much taller now than when I graduated.

I was such a happy kid growing-up; I always enjoyed making people laugh as well as a good joke or two. My teachers were very nice to me and I really enjoyed my early elementary years. I will never forget my grade 2 teacher, Miss. Marie Secondini. Miss. Secondini was an amazing teacher and she was so good to me. She enjoyed having me in her class, and made me feel so welcomed everyday. I remember that year she and my mom became good friends. My mom thought she was a fabulous teacher, and invited her to my

First Holy Communion party that spring. Miss. Secondini was a legend in Markham. Every parent wanted their child to be in her class. She taught grade 2 for the longest time, and my sister was also fortunate to have her as well when she was in grade 2. Miss. Secondini was known for her talents in playing the guitar and singing. For years she was our school's choir director. I enjoyed attending choir and singing with my friends. Once or twice a month we would sing at the 9 o'clock Children's Mass at our local parish. For elementary students we were pretty good. I however was not a good singer, but I just enjoyed being apart of the group, and besides in a group of 30 to 40 students, you were not able to hear me singing loudly. Thank God!

During elementary school I believe that it is important for children to have good teachers in order to be successful students. Students are so innocent at a young age, and it is crucial that they experience good teachers who will help them through their developing years. Grades 3 and 4 were also great years for me. I had terrific teachers both years, Mrs. Giardini and Mr. DeVries. I loved school during these years and was doing very well. I always had a smile on my face. Back then we really didn't deal with peer pressure, drugs etc., like many young children do today. My peers, teachers and educational assistances were very nice to me, and I would wake up each day eager to attend school.

Well time went on and I was coming close to the end of elementary school. Unfortunately the later parts of my elementary school days were very unpleasant from grade 5 onwards. Each year I felt like everyone was against me and nobody really understood me. I was constantly bullied by many male students, both younger and older than me, and whenever I would try to report them to my educational assistants, teachers or principal, my peers just made it look like I was a liar. I'll never forget in grade 8, I was being bullied in the boy's washroom by a grade 7 student. He kept asking me the dumbest questions like "What's wrong with you?" and "Are you gay?" This happened a few times, so I reported him to my EA. We got the principal involved, and eventually the three of us had a meeting. When she confronted the student, he denied doing this. He said to her that he thought I was stumbling over the toilet stall and he had asked me "Are you O.K.?" I could not believe this, it was his word against mine. I really could not wait until I left elementary school. It was a horrible experience for me. I constantly felt judged by staff and students, and could never defend myself whenever I was bullied.

I remember coming home many afternoons feeling so upset or sitting alone on a portable step during recess with tears running down my face. The one thing about having a disability is that we are easy targets. Just because we may have physical impairments, does not mean we lack cognitive abilities. However, people don't always see this in individuals like me. They look at the outside picture, and make assumptions based on our physical challenges. My mother has always taught me to never use the word hate, however, although there were some good times in elementary school, I can honestly say, I hated the later part of my elementary school days.

Not only was I dealing with bullies and teachers who did not understand me, like I mentioned before for many years I visited hospitals where I was referred to specialists and therapists who where supposed to help me improve my walking and speech. This was also a frustrating time for my parents and me. I remember going through a series of tests to see how they could improve my gait and speech. It was so embarrassing at times, going into hospital rooms and wearing very short shorts while my parents, doctors and therapists watched me walk. Now, the main concern in my walking was that my right foot constantly turns in. I tried my best (even to this very day) to make a conscientious effort to turn my foot out. Whenever I would go for testing the doctors could not see anything significantly wrong with my walking, and could not offer my parents and me any corrective surgeries. In terms of my speech therapy, I remember working with a therapist who was very particular about her methods. She wanted perfection from me, and this caused a lot of stress. I remember repeating words after her and never satisfying her. My mom would watch us working together and she could see me improving, and told her how frustrating it was for me. I realize my speech therapist was only helping me, however, when a child with a speech impairment is working hard, it is important to recognize their efforts and focus on the positives. She never encouraged me and rarely told me that I was doing a good job. So unfortunately my parents had to fire her, because I wasn't getting along with her, and after that I never really wanted to pursue speech therapy again.

Once a week, I would also work with my physiotherapist. She was a great help. Each week Maureen would come to my house and work on stretches with me, and teach my parents how to exercise with me as well. If you knew me from when I was really young, and see me now, there is a significant improvement on my physical abilities. I am so much stronger and can do a lot more on my own.

Growing up, physically I have had my fair share of challenges. However, among all the activities that I mentioned that I participated in as a child, I believe that it was downhill skiing that helped me the most with my walking abilities.

Each week my family would attend our ski club where my father would teach me how to ski. I skied with my dad's help for many years until I got older. However, skiing helped me build up my muscles, and my parents could see a significant improvement in the way I walked each year. I believe that skiing was the most effective therapy for me, and I wish I was able to continue to do it. Unfortunately, like all kids, I grew up, and it was hard for my dad to ski with me. Also I was no longer a fan of the cold weather, so I decided not to continue with skiing, and just focused on my education. Each year I brought home really good grades, and I truly enjoyed the academic side of school.

The later part of my elementary school days, I did not have much therapy. Maureen had moved on in her career, and I was focusing on getting out of elementary school. Nine years in the same school was more than I could handle. So many times I wanted to switch schools and attend a different school. A friend of my mom's was a teacher at St. Patrick's Catholic School, which is located beside our parish; and for years my mom and her talked about moving the kids over to her school. Looking back, I wish they had done this. The only reason why I stayed at Kateri Tekakwitha was because it was so close to home, and I was able to walk back and forth from school every day.

The last four years of elementary school I constantly felt judged, mainly by my teachers, educational assistants and administration. I could never explain myself in different situations, much like the washroom situation that I previously mentioned. So many times I would leave school early and go home sick as a dog, I used to think it was because our school was so warm and the heat would give me migraine headaches, but now looking back, I think it was stress related. I wanted to prove to them that I could handle the regular curriculum, but so many times I had failed. Some teachers thought I had a learning disability growing up, but it wasn't that at all. I had physical limitations, and I required assistance in class. As a qualified teacher, looking back on what I went through, I realize now that just because a student has physical limitations, should not have meant that they need to be isolated from their peers for a certain time of day, and placed in a special education class. But for years I went along with my teachers recommendations and did the best I could.

During grade 8, my special education teacher, had convinced my parents that I needed to continue to be educated in "special" classes. I remember my parents, teacher, principal and special education teacher getting together for meetings to discuss my academic future. I never understood why I wasn't involved in these meetings. I believe that all students with exceptionalities, as long as they understand what is going on, should have a say in their educational journey. After all it affects them. Well, I guess I didn't realize then what I know now. Therefore, I went along with what my teachers recommendations and I was placed in a small class learning basic level math and science, and not being challenged one bit. I tried to convince my teacher that I could do regular math, so she agreed to put me back in my grade 8 math class during their geometry unit. Well, picture this, a student with physical challenges who has poor fine motor skills trying to bisect a ninety degree angle with no educational support. I'm sorry but it's just not going to happen. Therefore, I finished elementary school taking a modified academic program.

Just because a student with physical challenges requires assistance with fine motor skills, does not mean that they need to be in a modified curriculum. I'm sure if my special education teacher knew that I am now a qualified teacher, with a college diploma and two university degrees she would be blown away. She had told my parents back when I was in grade 8 that I was not university material. How can anyone make that kind of assumption on a student at a young age? I can understand if a student was not performing at all, but I was getting very good grades. I believe that teachers need to help students with exceptionalities, celebrate their uniqueness and guide them properly to achieve all that they can in life. I can't speak for others, but when someone tells me that "I can't" do something; it makes me want to work even harder to prove them wrong. There were some highlights in grade 8 that year. My class took many great trips that I was able to participate in like, Canada's Wonderland, Pleasure Valley, and our big graduation trip to Ottawa. This was an amazing trip for my peers and myself. My dad came with me as an extra parent chaperon and we all stayed in a five-star hotel, the Chateau Laurier. We were given the opportunity to tour Ottawa, and visit many historical sites, like Parliament Hill and Rideau Canal. It was so much fun. I really enjoyed the extra curricular activities in grade 8. This year was also significant for my peers and me, as we were preparing for our Sacrament of Confirmation. This was very important for me, preparing for this sacrament made me feel closer to God and my faith. However, I soon found out that I could not receive this sacrament because I had already done so when I was baptized.

When my parents were married, they had their wedding in my dad's Church, which was Greek Orthodox. They did this to please my dad's family. In the Greek Church it is customary for the best man and his wife to baptize the couples first born child. Since there were complications at the time I was born, my parents didn't worry too much about which church I was baptized in, and therefore allowed my Godparents to baptize me in their church. My parents had started attending Mass at the Greek Orthodox church early on in their marriage, however they did not find happiness there; therefore my mother brought us back to the church where she had been raised, which was the Roman Catholic tradition. Since both faiths have many similarities, I was able to participate in the Catholic Church.

When a child is baptized in the Greek Church, they receive the sacraments of initiation at the same time, Baptism, Holy Communion and Confirmation. This was disappointing for me, because at this point in my life I was an active member of the Catholic Church and I wanted to be confirmed as a Catholic. My philosophy is that Baptism is a decision that parents make for their children, and Confirmation should be your choice when you are older. I attended Mass every week, and still do to this very day. I was also involved in youth group with my friends. Church life was (and still is) very important to me. The year of what was supposed to be my Confirmation; my parish priest arranged a meeting for my parents and myself to speak with the Archbishop. This was important, because he was going to explain to me why I could not be confirmed twice. After speaking with the Archbishop, he explained to me how both religions are very similar, and the Catholic Church recognized my Baptism and Confirmation and you cannot receive these sacraments more then once in your life. Still I felt I had to do something, because my whole life I had been brought up as a Roman Catholic and wanted to be a part of this important milestone of my religious life. Although my original Baptism could not be reversed, the Archbishop did allow me to reaffirm my faith and renew my Baptismal promises in the Catholic Church. This was a significant time in my life, as it brought me closer to God and to the Church.

This event in my life made me feel like an important member of the Church and on my Confirmation day, I could feel the Holy Spirit enter into me in a miraculous way, and I believe His Spirit has in fact been guiding me all these years. His Spirit has also helped me become the strong individual that I am today. Without my faith in God I would not be where I am today. With God's Grace along with the guidance of the Holy Spirit, I have overcome many challenges in life and have tackled numerous obstacles that some people doubted I could ever accomplish.

That year my classmates and I had to choose a sponsor to Confirm us. I was looking forward to this for many years, because I had known who my sponsor was going to be. In my early elementary days we had met a wonderful family, the Titanic's. Paul, Linda and their children David and Kristy were like our extended family members. We did so much together. We attended Mass together, invited one another over for dinners, and took a few trips together. We were like one big happy family. Their son David, who I ended up sponsoring for his Confirmation, is a big hockey fan. For years I would go watch him play in tournaments and games all over Ontario. People began to think I was Paul and Linda's oldest son. I remember one game it was just Paul, David and myself. After the game I was waiting for them to come out of the change room and one of the hockey dads approached me. He came up to me and said "Hey Pete, where's you're Dad?" I looked at him and said "at home." He gave me the strangest look, and said "Your Dad, Paul?" I felt embarrassed and didn't want to correct him, so I said, "Oh that Dad, he's in the change room". I remember on the way home telling Paul that story, and we had a good chuckle.

Paul and I have had a special friendship over the years, and I chose him to be my Confirmation sponsor that year because he was so good to me. He always included me in activities with his family and always takes the time to see how everything is going for me. For many years they came to our cottage where we spent a week boating, tubing and enjoying each others company. I remember one year we took a trip out east. Both families embarked on a two week road trip where we visited eastern Canada. We visited Quebec, Prince Edward Island, New Brunswick and Nova Scotia. It was so much fun and we all got along so well. It was an amazing trip and a true test of our friendship. Not many people can spend as much time as we have over the years, take a trip together where we shared a 5 bedroom house, and still be friends. To this very day, we are still great friends and I constantly rely on my sponsor for guidance, support and love. He is a remarkable man; my family and I are so fortunate to have Mr. T (that's what I call him) and his family in our lives. Our friendship continues to grow year after year.

As I mentioned before, when I was getting ready to graduate from elementary school that year the same year as my Confirmation, my special education teacher had little faith in my academic performance and persuaded my parents to enrol me in basic level classes for my grade 9 core subjects: English, History, Math as well as Science. My special education teacher recommended and convinced my parents that this was the best thing for me without consulting the most important person, *me*. I graduated from elementary school in June of 1998 and I was so happy to get out of that school. Although there were some teachers that I was going to miss as well as many wonderful memories, I was more than ready to move on in life and begin my next chapter.

That June as I was about to graduate, my grandparents informed me that they were not going to be able to attend the graduation ceremony because they had some business to take care of in Florida. I was a little disappointed. However, as a gift, they bought me a plane ticket to Florida, so that I could spend the summer down south with them. I was so excited. I remember graduation night as if it were yesterday. We had the ceremony and dinner at St. Patrick's Church; it was a fun evening, and a great way to end my elementary school journey. The following day I left for Florida. It was my first time on an airplane by myself. I was so excited to see my grandparents. For my graduation one of my mom's good friends who I call Ciotka Irene, which means Auntie Irene in Polish, gave me a leather journal for my trip. Each day she had asked me to write in my journal what I had done with my grandparents. I had so much fun that summer with my grandparents. My grandfather spent most of his days building the family plaza, and my grandmother and I spent our day's together, shopping, baking, visiting friends and enjoying the sun as well as each others company.

That summer I surprised my grandmother with a birthday party. It wasn't a significant year; she was turning 64-years-old. I just wanted to surprise her and thank her for taking care of me. Her friends helped me throw the party and we told my grandma the party was for one of their mutual friends. Now, whenever you tell my grandmother there is a party, she always wants to get involved. It was so hard not to tell her that the party was for her. So she ended up making the main course meal, which was lasagne. Looking back now, it was actually pretty comical. Here my grandmother was walking in to her own surprise party with a tray of lasagne. She is the best grandmother any grandchild could ask for. My sister, cousins and myself, are so lucky to have terrific grandparents.

The summer was flying by, and even though I was enjoying my time in Florida, I wanted to go home. I remember calling my mom and telling her that I was home sick. She told me to hang in because they were coming down in August. Well as it turned out, they ended up coming down earlier than planned and we spent the rest of the summer as a family in Florida. It was a great trip and we left the end of August and drove home. High school was just around the corner.

HIGH SCHOOL: MY FONDEST EDUCATION EXPERIENCES

Sooner than later I found myself in the hallways of St. Brother Andre Catholic High School, formerly known as Brother Andre Catholic High School. Like all grade nine's I was anxious about high school. I had the usual grade nine jitters. Back then I thought that the school was huge, and I was worried about going from class to class, making new friends, and doing well academically. However, high school was nothing like I expected. It was a great time, and perhaps my favourite time in life. I enjoyed having different teachers and meeting new friends. One of the highlights of high school for me was seeing Mrs. Badali again. She introduced me to the other EAs and told me that I was going to love high school; it was going to be a wonderful experience.

Boy was she right. High school was an amazing time for me. Everyone was so friendly and my teachers were fantastic. I enjoyed having different classes and not being in the same classroom all day. The only downside to high school was the academic side of grade 9. It wasn't all that I had expected. Growing up, I had always enjoyed the math and science part of school, but English wasn't my forte. However, being in the modified program I ended up getting a 93 per cent as a midterm mark in English. Now what does that tell you? I'm too smart? No, it simply means that I wasn't being challenged enough. Therefore after grade nine I decided to take control of my own academic career. It was time for me to make my own path in life. I spoke to my guidance counsellor that year, and as a result of my determination, in grade 10 I took general level courses with a few advanced level courses.

Back then the curriculum consisted of three levels of learning; basic, general and advanced. Basic level courses prepared students for the workforce, general level course were designed for college-bound students and advanced level courses prepared students for university life. And guess what? Not only did I do well in the general level courses, I made the honour roll that year. Therefore, I told my guidance counsellor I needed to take advanced level courses in grades 11 and onwards. After four years of high school I graduated in grade 12 with OAC courses as well. At that time the province of Ontario had OAC, which was formally known as grade 13.

The summer after grade 9, my family had planned a trip to Europe. I was looking forward to this all year. We went with some family friends, and decided to spend a week on a cruise, visiting three countries and a week on an island. We visited Italy, France, Spain, and the second week on the island of Majorca, which is off the eastern coast of Spain. It was a great trip; my parents brought my wheelchair with us which allowed us to see so many historical sites. This was such a rich experience. I learned so much about these three countries and I hope I have the opportunity to visit more European countries in the future. I would love to visit Greece where my dad was born, as well as England and Paris as I have friends who live in both of these places. We did not get a chance to see Paris when we were in France.

As the years went on in high school, each year I accomplished so much, and fell in love with a new passion.

I was very involved in high school, and tried to participate in extracurricular activities as much as I could. In grade 10 I took a hospitality class. This was the only class where I had an EA as oppose to a peer helper. Like I mentioned above, EAs are hired by the Boards, where as peer helpers are students within the school who help other students with exceptionalities while earning a credit. I enjoyed working in the kitchen and helping my peers prepare meals for the school restaurant. Each week we would rotate in the kitchen and work on preparing different courses of the daily lunch menu. That semester I fell in love with baking and found my knack in baking dinner rolls for the school restaurant. My bread was a legend in the school community. Word had got out that I was in charge of baking the restaurant's dinner rolls, and so many staff members complemented me on how good my dinner rolls tasted.

I remember the following semester I was no longer enrolled in hospitality, so I continued going into the kitchen every morning at 7:30 to prepare the dough for the dinner rolls. No one asked me to do this; I just took it upon myself to help out. The hospitality teachers, Mr. Sheridan, and Mr. Cook, (yes that is his real last name) were so impressed with me, and I ended up winning the Casey Choice Award for my hard work and dedication. This weekly award was a program at my high school that awarded one student for his or her dedication or doing something of significance to better the school community. I remember my name was posted on the school's outdoor board for the entire community to see. It was such a great honour.

Grade 10 was a wonderful year. I finished off the year with honours, and had planned my grade 11 year in the advanced level program. I was doing very well in school and had a dream of going to university in my future. In grade 11 this was the year when I fell in love with fitness. I enrolled in a fitness and weight training course, my teacher Ms. Ann Turrin, was very supportive of me, and encouraged me to be active in class. The academic side of grade 11 was a bit challenging; however, I enjoyed the challenge and being enrolled in academic courses made me feel very good about myself as it helped me improve my academic abilities and challenge myself academically.

That year I was passing all of my courses and getting pretty decent grades. It is important for students to remember that school should not be all about the grades. School should be about challenging ourselves to do well and continue succeeding. Teachers need to make students aware that school is not a competition. The only person students should compete against is themselves and work hard each year to improve their academic abilities. One way this can be done is for teachers to begin each year or semester, by having their students write down a mark in which they hope to achieve in a specific course. This way student can stay focus on their goal and work hard to earn the grade that they are striving for.

Grade 11 was a wonderful year for me. I remember we had four foreign exchange students visit my high school for the year. Three of the girls were from Columbia (which is a country in the northern part of South America) and the fourth girl was from Paris, France. They were so much fun to hang around with and treated me like their brother. I'll never forget for my 17th birthday, the Columbian girls sang me "Happy Birthday" in Spanish during our fitness class; it was so cool hanging out with them. They were living with a family in my neighbourhood, and many times we would walk home from school together. We kept in touch for many years after they left Canada. Unfortunately their e-mail addresses have changed and we lost contact. I miss them so much and I hope they are all doing well.

The years flew by fast and I was now a high school senior. That year I fell in love with writing. I was a writer for the school paper and I was also taking a grade 13 writing course. I was a pretty good writer. One of my articles had even won a recognition award. After finding a love for newspaper writing I decided to attend college the following year where I wanted to study Journalism-Print. I graduated from high school in 2002 with two awards, the Physical Education and Health award and the Jean Vanier award. For those of you who do not know who Jean Vanier is, let me tell you. Jean Vanier is a Canadian Catholic philosopher, humanitarian and the founder of L'Arche. L'Arche is an international organization which creates communities where people with developmental disabilities and those who assist them share life together.

I was so happy to have won this award. I had enjoyed working with other students with exceptionalities that year, and was enrolled in a peer helping class where I worked with a young girl, who had autism spectrum disorder. This was a wonderful opportunity, and I would encourage all high school students to take peer helping at least once before they graduate. I really enjoyed working with her and helping her develop her skills on a daily basis. Working as a peer helper in the special education department was a wonderful experience for me. This taught me so much about how individuals live with autism and what gifts they can bring to any community. Back then, getting into teaching was not on my radar, however, I really enjoyed working as a peer helper in the special education department, and making a difference in the lives of others.

That same year on graduation night I also had won the physical and health education award, which was even a bigger honour for me as I really enjoyed participating in all of my phys-ed classes over the years. Back then phys-ed was only mandatory for students to take in grades 9 and 10. However, I enjoyed the courses so much that I took it all four years of high school. I remember in my grade twelve fitness class our final project was to design a fitness circuit for the entire class and it had to last one full period. I partnered up with a classmate and started thinking about what to do. Unfortunately my partner did not get involved at all and I ended up putting the entire circuit together myself and teaching it to the class, with the help from my peer helper. I did a great job and ended up getting an A on the assignment. My phys-ed teacher, Mr. John Spicer, was very impressed with me, and to this day I have a feeling that he was the teacher who nominated me for the phys-ed award when I graduated.

* * *

I have come across many wonderful teachers who have inspired me to do my best in any academic performance. In particular, when I was in high school I came across a number of tremendous teachers, who have encouraged me to do my best in life. Mr. Spicer was one of my favorite teachers growing up. He believed that I could accomplish anything in life. He always tells me to this very day how he uses me as an example of perseverance and determination in his physical education classes. I remember one day in class some students were slacking off, and he was so mad. He said to them, "look at Peter, if he can do it, then you guys should have no excuses." I was so honoured and scared at the same time. I remember thinking, boy these guys are going to beat me up after school.

However, nothing happened to me and I continued working hard in my physical education class.

Mr. Spicer is the kind of teacher who makes learning enjoyable. When I eventually obtain a teaching position, I want to make sure that I am just like Mr. Spicer. He is a passionate teacher who encourages his students to participate in their physical education classes as much as possible. As an individual with a physical disability, Mr. Spicer made me feel like a valuable student who was always welcomed in his class. Students enjoy attending his classes and working hard. I always made sure that I was a diligent student in his phys-ed classes so that he would know that I was a dedicated student. Like myself, Mr. Spicer believes that all students should be equal members of the classroom environment, no matter what challenges he or she may face. His enthusiasm for teaching as well as student success clearly depicts what kind of individual he is. After having been taught my Mr. Spicer, I am able to remember the positive motivation I received as his student. As an aspiring teacher, I can learn from this amazing individual, and make sure that my future classroom will be an inviting atmosphere that welcomes all students, with all kinds of abilities and disabilities. I have realized that when your students see their teacher showing interest in who they are and what they choose to study, then they will model their teacher and strive for academic achievement. Mr. Spicer's passion for teaching and acceptance for all students, tells me a great deal about his identity and integrity. This also tells me that he is an individual who cares about his students, and he doesn't look at teaching as just a job, but rather a calling. I truly believe that God has called Mr. Spicer to pursue a vocation in teaching, so that he can continue to touch the lives of so many young individuals, just like he has touched mine.

So many teachers I have met admit that it was not the methods they learned in teacher's college that enabled them to become excellent teachers, but rather what they learned about people in their on-the-job experience. One may have all the methodology correctly engaged and still not connect with the students. Good teachers are people persons; excellent teachers are confident persons. They trust themselves, are true to themselves, and are not afraid to go out on a limb for the welfare of the students they encounter in their everyday classroom experience. To be an excellent teacher, communication skills is so vital. I must first see the needs and concerns of my students, before I teach any subject. I must take the student where they are and not where I might wish them to be. Some teachers worry so much about covering the curriculum that they do so at any cost to the student. This might be in pilling on the work or manipulating performance records in order to make themselves look good. An excellent teacher takes risks, shares himself or herself at a personal and often vulnerable level. He or she knows that at times they will be criticized, that everyone will not necessarily like them. They know they are not running a popularity contest for "teacher of the year". This same excellent teacher is guided chiefly by what is best for this student, not making carbon copies of everyone who passes through his classroom. This teacher realizes that their students before them may have entered their classroom with not enough to eat, or addiction problems, or difficult home situations, and perhaps this student may have other things on his agenda besides their studies.

That year I had mixed emotions about leaving high school. I could have stayed one more semester and completed my OAC courses, but for some strange reason, something was telling me that it was time to move on. My parents had planned a big party for me that spring. It was a party to celebrate my 18th birthday as well as my high school graduation. We had so many people there. My mom surprised me and invited Uncle Jimmy and his family. It was so great seeing them, as I didn't really see them that often. However, looking back now I wish I had spent more time with my uncle. The day of my party, Sunday, June 9th, 2002 was the last time I saw him. I remember during the summer he had called us and asked me if he could speak with either of my parents. Unfortunately they were not home at the time. My parents tried to call him back, but had no luck connecting with him.

He and his wife were having some problems and had separated that year. I remember we had gone away that August to Florida and upon our return home, we found out that my uncle had passed away. He had a heart attack while water skiing at his cottage. I was devastated and to this very day I still miss him so much. Perhaps he has been my guardian angel who has been guiding me through my life since then.

MY POST-SECONDARY JOURNEY BEGINS

During my final semester of high school I was accepted at Durham College in Oshawa, Ontario, where I studied Journalism-Print. My dream was to become a well-known writer for a major newspaper company. I began my first year and lived away from home on campus. This was a new journey for me and it was very challenging. I remember the first few weeks living on campus was so new to me. I choose to live in residence on my own. I was worried about having a roommate. Within the first month of school I managed to carry a full course load in school while struggling to live by myself. Although my parents were there to help me out, I had my ups and downs. One night I managed to choke on a piece of pineapple and was taken by an ambulance to Oshawa General Hospital. It was a cold and stormy winter night, my dad wasn't home and my mom drove from Markham to the hospital to make sure I was alright. I just love my parents; they are the most loving individuals I know. They are always there to help me and make sure I am doing all that I can to succeed. After my little choking incident I later went for testing, where I found out I had acid reflex. I was put on medication which has helped a great deal to this very day.

My parents have always been there for me, through thick and thin. My mom is a wonderful woman who gave up her career in advertising, to stay home to raise my sister and me. She is always there for me and is constantly supporting me in all that I do. My dad, being a teacher, has always been there to help me whenever I needed help with school, friends, dealing with my teachers or any roadblock in life. They have both loved me unconditionally, and want nothing but the best for my sister and me. My parents look at my sister and me as God's children, and He has chosen them to be our "adopted" earth parents. Over the years they have been there to wipe our tears, celebrate our achievements and guide us along the right path in live. They raised us in the Catholic faith, and taught us that with God's grace, anything in life is possible. Although my sister and I have done our fair share of disappointing them at times, we are a loving and caring family who look out for each other and always have each other's best interests at heart.

My second year of college was much better. At the post-secondary level of education, educational assistants are not provided to students. My disability advisor, Linda Lyons recommended that I apply for government funding to access disability grants. Unfortunately due to my parents combined annual income I was denied OSAP, (OSAP stands for Ontario Student Assistant Program). Each year if you qualify, the federal and/or provincial funding, the government will give students either loans or grants, or in some cases a combination of both, to help fund your academic expenses. However, since I was denied funding, Linda encouraged me to write a letter to the college's financial aid office explaining my dilemma, and what I needed the funding for. I told them that in order to be successful in Journalism-Print program, I required assistants and technology to help me succeed. I requested a new computer, a digital camera, and educational assistants. As a journalist, we needed to write stories, interview people and take photographs to go with our articles. Having a helping hand was essential for my success in the program. Fortunately I was granted $10,000 to cover these expenses. I was so grateful and had a very successful year. Just because I could handle myself academically, physically I require assistance, and this funding was so important and with the help I received this allowed me to be very successful.

That summer I came home and worked at my parish for the second summer in a row. This was a great opportunity for me. It allowed me to work with a few friends from my youth group days; we had so much fun working together. My friends were in charge of running the Bible youth day camp and I worked in the office as an assistant. I did work for both the Church and the camp. I enjoyed going to work each day. Not many students have the opportunity to work in God's House. This experience brought me even closer to my Church community and my faith.

Now my college program was a two-year program; however I was taking a reduced course load, which meant that I had an extra year to complete the program. That summer I had saved enough money from my job to pay for my tuition. I found out that GO Transit had opened a route from Unionville, Ontario, which is a town not too far from where I was living in Markham. I had inquired about this before my final year started, and one of the college staff members, looked into this for me, and Go Transit ended up opening the bus route. This bus route went straight to my campus in Oshawa. I was so grateful to live back at home for my final year and complete my diploma. All was going well for me that year. My grades were improving and I was publishing weekly articles in the school *Chronicle*, which was our school's paper. I even made the honour roll that year.

When life seemed like it was going well I hit a minor road block. I ran into some problems with one of my bus drivers. He was giving me a hard time, as he told me that it was not his responsibility to help me on and off the bus with my walker. This was so stressful for me, and I did not have the time to deal with this. Although I did not have him for every ride, the times that I did made it very uncomfortable. I will never forget, on the GO buses they have a sign that indicates where they are going. It usually said "Unionville or Kennedy GO Station". One day the bus pulled up and the sign read "Special". I was thinking *what does this mean?* So I asked the driver if he was going to Kennedy, and he said "no". Therefore I had to wait for the next bus. Meanwhile, he did drive to Kennedy station where my dad always met me after work. My dad didn't see me get off the bus, so he approached the driver to see where I was. The driver then lied to him and said that I was not at the bus stop in Oshawa. I finally caught the next bus, an hour later, which happened to be the last bus out. When I arrived to the station my dad asked what had happened. I explained the situation to him, which led to us contacting the Go Transit head office. Now since bus drivers are unionized, we had a hard time getting rid of this driver. Fortunately they ended up changing his route and the other drivers were very helpful.

After three years of hard work and having to repeat only one course, I graduated from Durham College with my diploma. My parents were so proud of me. I even completed a seven week internship at Toronto Community News, where I published weekly articles in local Toronto newspapers. This was a great experience for me as I got to see first-hand how things ran inside a newsroom. I volunteered there five-days-a-week, and each day was given a different assignment. It was so much fun; family and friends would call me whenever they saw my name in their local paper. I felt like a movie star!

That spring at my college graduation I must have had the largest number of guests come to see me receive my diploma. My parents, my maternal grandparents, sister, my confirmation sponsor and his wife, Linda, and my favorite Aunt Josie were all there to celebrate my success and see me graduate. It was a wonderful and memorable day. After graduation, this is where the job hunting began. That spring I was unsuccessful at finding employment, so I volunteered at my high school in their special education department. I immediately fell in love with teaching and working alongside students with exceptionalities. Therefore, I decided that teaching was the career path I wanted to pursue. I found out I needed an undergraduate degree and then an education degree, so I had applied to York University that year just in case, and ended up accepting their offer of enrollment. I started at York the same year as my sister, and let me tell you, I could not have done this with out her.

I COULD HAVE NEVER MADE IT THIS FAR WITHOUT MY SISTER

Before I continue talking about my journey, let me take the time to introduce you to my sister. Stephanie Nicole Mitskinis was born on March 11th, 1987. I was so happy when my parents brought her home. They told me that she was my sister, all mine. I enjoyed holding her, kissing her and playing with her. She was and still is the highlight of my life; the apple of my eye. Until she turned two, that is. Many of you think the term "terrible twos" is just a saying; well let me be the first to tell you, my sister was no angel at that age, she was a piece of work. She was into everything. She never learned to walk, and no, she did not have cerebral palsy, all she could do was run. Although my parents were in the best physical shape of their lives, while running after her, Stephanie was a handful. But like all children she grew up into the most spunky, beautiful young lady that I am proud to call my sister. The same year that I graduated from Durham College, she too graduated from high school, and together we attended York University the following September. Steph was a great help, we had two courses together in our first year where she shared her notes with me, and we traveled together to and from school on the GO Bus. She was so helpful and I am grateful that she decided to attend a local university and live at home.

HOW I GOT THROUGH THE UPS AND DOWNS OF UNIVERSITY

My first year of university was a challenge. Although I passed all of my courses I was a bit stressed and almost decided to quit. My parents talked me into sticking it through and I finished off my first year successfully. I took courses on a part time bases, however, because of my disability I was considered a full time student. This was a blessing because this meant I qualified for student loans and grants. My parents had helped me out financially in college, but now it was my turn to take care of my educational expenses. Each year I found out more ways to apply for bursaries and scholarships which allowed me to hire tutors and note takers. I was so grateful for their financial assistance. Every year before the next school year began I advertised on facebook to hire note takers to help me out. With funding from the university I was able to pay them and I was so happy with the support I received.

As the years moved on, university life improved for me. I was doing really well and passing all of my courses. I was able to hold down summer jobs which helped me pay for my education and I was able to focus on my studies during the school year. My Confirmation sponsor, who I mentioned before, had started a hockey camp back when I was in high school, and each summer he hired me to work as a registration clerk during the weeks that the camps were running. I was also given the opportunity to work at my parish, Church of St. Patrick's two summers in a row as an office assistant. One summer I was given the chance to volunteer for an organization known as Character Community. I volunteered for the Executive Director whose office happened to be located in the York Catholic District School Board. This unpaid internship led me to paid positions within the Board that summer. I was very grateful for this. Unfortunately, due to cutbacks I was not able to return to the Board the following summer. However, that summer I met many people in the school board, and was given a number of assignments in various departments. When my supervisors and other staff members began to know who I was, and found out my ambitions for becoming a teacher, they were very supportive and encouraged me to pursue my educational dreams. This gave me the strength and determination to continue my pursuit to be a teacher.

Time went on and as each school year ended in April I found myself volunteering in the special education department at St. Brother Andre C.H.S in Markham. I worked with the department head, Zita Van Oosten. Mrs. Van Oosten was my special education teacher in high school, and she always enjoys whenever I volunteer my time at the school. Through my volunteer experiences, this is where I began to realize that I wanted to become a special education teacher just like her. I had worked with a variety of students that year who had many different exceptionalities. This was a wonderful experience and really opened my eyes to what it would be like to be a special education teacher. I remember at the end of June I told my parents that I really enjoyed my volunteer experience, and teaching was the path that I wanted to pursue.

The following September I continued on at York University and I was told by my student advisor that if I wanted to attend teacher's college, I needed to take two subjects that I could eventually teach. Now, since I wanted to work in special education, I found out that this is not offered in university, I would have to take additional qualification courses once I graduated from teachers college. Therefore, I decided to study Religious Studies and Geography. I was a very dedicated student in university, although I didn't make the honour roll in university, I did manage to do really well. I completed my Bachelor of Arts degree in three and a half years. During this time I had taken one semester off where I spent most of it in Florida with my maternal grandparents, I really enjoyed spending time with them in Florida. University was challenging for me, I was a bit overwhelmed during my third year and dropped my second semester courses. This really helped me recharge myself, and motivated me to return to school.

Like I mentioned before, my grandparents are amazing people and without their love, support and spiritual guidance I would not be where I am today. My grandmother and I have a special bond. I keep telling her that she is very lucky, because no 28-year-old would be OK with spending as much time with them as I do. To this day if I get busy with job hunting, volunteering, or with my commitment at my church as an RCIA sponsor, and forget to call them, I hear about it. My sister and I call it the grandparent guilt-trip and boy are they good at it. Growing up with a physical disability my grandmother has always said that I am a "gift from God". When I was a young boy, she brought me to a place called Our Lady of Fatima Shrine, which is in Lewiston, New York. This place is a religious site that many people visit and pray. One of their religious monuments that I remember is a long set of concrete stairs that people climb while reciting the rosary. Now, for those of you who are not Catholic, the rosary is a traditional Catholic devotion. The term symbolizes the prayer beads used to count the series of prayers, mainly the Lord's Prayer and Hail Mary's, that make up the rosary.

This shrine has become a place of natural beauty, art, communal prayer and faith-renewal to thousands who visit each year. To this very day my grandmother tells everyone the story of how when we visited this place, I began to walk independently shortly after. My grandmother and I believe that it was with the help of the Virgin Mary and God's grace, that I have overcome this challenge in life. I am so fortunate to have my grandparents and even though they are still fairly young, I pray that God continues to keep them strong and healthy.

In my third year at York University I had officially met a lady by the name of Terri Penny. We had been going to the same parish, St. Patrick's, for many year, but had not met. She was attending Niagara University at the time and studying to become a high school teacher. When Terri found out about my ambitions in becoming a teacher as well, she immediately told me about her program and introduced me to Tom Donovan, who is the Director of the Niagara University education program in Ontario. I had also met a number of faculty members including Dr. Peter Cowden, who is a professor at the university. It was here that I learned a great deal about their program, and was encouraged by the faculty to apply.

This program seemed perfect for me. It was spread out over three semesters, and the practice teaching experiences were set up gradually. This meant that in our first semester we participated in an observation placement, where we asked to job shadow a teacher. The second semester we were to partake in a Teaching Assistantship, where we helped in a classroom and worked with the teacher. Finally, the last semester was our teaching placements, where we were to work with a teacher and teach their courses on a fulltime bases. I really liked layout of the program because it gradually prepared teacher candidates for the teaching profession. After learning about the program I submitted my application and I was looking forward to attending the following year.

When I came back home from Florida I returned to York University. I took one course during the spring semester and enough courses the following year to graduate in June of 2009. Just like my college graduation, this graduation was just as special for me, maybe even more. That spring before graduation my sister and I were both accepted to the Niagara University teaching program.

I attended an information session at Niagara University with my mom and sister and it was there that I learned more about the program. The program looked very interesting, it was an American school that was based in Ontario and we were told that this program was very unique because of the amount of in-class practice teaching experience teacher candidates received. Although the tuition fee was very expensive I told my parents that I would save my money because this is what I really wanted to do for myself. That year I received bursaries and scholarships, and along with my graduation gifts, I had saved $14,000; almost enough to pay for my tuition fee.

My sister and I were so excited to graduate and continue our final educational journey. During that same time our mom was about to turn 50, (but let's keep that between you and me). I decided I wanted to surprise her with a birthday party, because she deserved it. So I conspired with one of her good friends, Janet, to help my sister, my dad and I throw her a big birthday bash. It was a huge success, and to top it off, I surprised everyone and had my mom's best friend from Texas fly in to celebrate.

WHO IS KATE RYAN?

Again I am going to side track here and introduce to you another important person in my life. Her name is Kate Ryan, but we Canadians refer to her as Kathy. Kathy is my mom's best friend and mine as well. People used to think that she and my mom were separated at birth because of their similar characteristics. They both have an awesome sense of humor, (but that's a book in itself), loving qualities, and they are both exceptional moms. Kathy is an American who was born in a little town called Tonawanda, which is near Buffalo, New York. Now I can't give you Kathy's life story, but I'll tell you what I do know about this wonderful person. She grew up in Anaheim, California and later moved to Salt Lake City, Utah. She spent many years in Utah where she attended university and met her first husband, Peter, who happened to be Canadian. After university they were married and had their first daughter, Trisha. A few years after Trisha was born Peter was transferred to Toronto, Canada where they ended up becoming our neighbors. To this day I am so grateful for this. Our families were so close during the years they lived here. When Kathy and my mom first met, people used to think they were sisters. They actually kind of resembled each other back then.

We did so much together; Kathy was and still is my hero, role model and friend. I often think of her as one of my aunts. Growing up with Kathy and her family, our families spent a great deal of time together. We had dinners at each other's homes, celebrated birthdays together and the kids got along very well. My mom always told me that as children she would never leave my sister and me with anyone but my grandparents, mainly because I required a lot of help and my sister was a handful. She always tells me the story of when she turned 30, Kathy forced her to go out for dinner with my dad to celebrate. That night Kathy came over and kidnapped my sister and me, so that my parents could have a night to themselves. This story always puts a smile on my face, because it reminds me of who Kathy really is. She is a wonderful friend, mother, sister and daughter. Those who know her are so blessed to have her in their lives, I know that I am. For those who don't know her, I suggest you get to know her. I can only speak for myself, but knowing Kathy and having her in my life is truly a blessing from God. If I had never met her, I would definitely have an empty void in my life. She always tells me of how grateful she is of our friendship, and how we will be friends for eternity.

Unfortunately, Kathy's husband was relocated to Texas, and they ended up moving there over twenty years ago. I miss them so much, but thanks to Internet, phones and airplanes we manage to keep in touch. I was actually there the summer of my 27th birthday, celebrating with Kathy and her family. This goes to show you what kind of person she is. Despite my disability I was able to fly down there on my own and spend six wonderful days with them.

I'm getting ahead of myself here. The same year of my mom's 50th birthday, Kathy along with her husband Jim and son Nick, flew to Toronto to celebrate both my sister and my university graduation. Unfortunately I did not have enough tickets for all three to attend our graduation ceremony, but Kathy was there cheering me on. I will never forget when

I went up on stage to receive my degree everyone in my family was cheering for me, but all I heard was "Way to go Peter, Wahoo!!" and guess who it was? Yes, it was Kathy. In an auditorium of probably 2000 people, I could hear Kathy cheering me on.

Kathy is an inspiration to me. For many years she was a single mom to her four wonderful children, Trish, Brook, Kimberly and Nicholas. As a single mom, Kathy managed to hold down a full-time job and her own house while taking care of her children and attending university. Kathy is a very intelligent person. She has received her undergraduate degree, as well as her master's degree. Knowing what she has gone through and what obstacles she has overcome and accomplished in life, has inspired me to be successful just like her.

I have to mention Kathy's son, Nick in my story. This young man is truly amazing. He is the kind of son any mother would want, and a brother that I wish I had. Nick is awesome. When his family and he came to Toronto to celebrate Stephanie and my graduation, it was the first time we had met him. We knew of Nick since the day he was born, and seen him grow up through Christmas card photos in the mail, but we had not officially met. He is truly a smart individual and the kind of student any teacher would want in his classroom. Nick is very accepting of people, and when I first met him he was so kind to me. He was able to look pass my disability and treat me with love, admiration and respect. If I could have an entire classroom filled with students who had Nick's charming personality and character, I would be the luckiest teacher in the world.

On the day of my graduation his family had given my sister and me a very generous gift. When Nick saw us opening our gifts, he was upset that he did not have a card of his own to give us. The following day before we were headed north to take them to our cottage, Nick made his mom drive him to Wal-Mart to buy a card for my sister and me. When he gave me my card, I opened it and could not believe what I saw; inside was $10 from him and a beautiful note that read:

Dear Peter, I hope you had a fantastic day. I am very sorry that this card is late, but either way I send the most of my love. You are a great friend; you are kind, trustworthy, loyal, helpful and friendly. I can't even explain how much of an inspiration you are to me. Congrats on graduating from college. Love Always, Nick.

I was so surprised and happy. I had only officially met him 24 hours ago and his words have touched me to this very day. I absolutely love Nick, and I envy his teachers who have the opportunity to work with him each day. I never told any one, but I secretly e-mailed his principal in McKinney, Texas, where he lives, to see if I could get a teaching job at his school, however, I was unsuccessful.

Nick is a football player and last year he had an important game in Texas. He wanted to win so badly. Therefore, for good luck he wrote my name around his wrist band, said nothing to his mom and went off to his game. That night I received a Facebook message from Kathy that said,

"Peter—Nick got his wrists wrapped for the football game and dedicated his game to you...And they won! Wish you could have been there!"

This made my day. Nick is such a special friend.

Kathy's husband Jim is also a great friend of mine and I am so lucky to have met him. Whenever I am with Jim we have amazing conversations and I enjoy our time together. I have shared many personal stories with him about me. Jim is a very religious and spiritual man; he has a close relationship with God, and has taught me so much about his faith. Jim is like no other person I've ever meet, he is kind-hearted, loving, compassionate and a great friend to many. I look forward to each time I spend with Kate, Jim and Nick.

My final year at York University was very successful. I was very dedicated and worked with a tutor who helped me with my major assignments. While attending university, formal essay writing was not my forte. I was known to be an excellent writer; I just needed extra help with formulating my ideas, and developing proper academic papers. I had hired a lady from my parish by the name of Jean Howard. I have known Jean for many years as her daughter and I both attended both elementary and secondary school together. Jean and I would work together each week on my assignments. She is a wonderful person and a great help. Like many students I found university challenging, but knowing that I wanted to become a teacher helped me to stay focused on my dream and continue on the road of success.

MY SUCCESS IN TEACHERS COLLEGE

Education is a key component in all our lives today, and no matter what kind of student we are, it is important to continue achieving our goals and work hard at becoming successful. Education is one of many things that cannot be taken away from us. Living in a country like Canada we are all very blessed to be given the opportunities and freedom to pursue education. We often take this for granted as many other countries deny this right to women, as well as those who have exceptionalities experience discrimination. Racial prejudices have always been part of our society for hundreds of years. In the Western world we are all given equal opportunities, no matter our race, ethnicity, abilities, gender, religion, etc. Today more and more students are pursuing their post-secondary education two and three times over. I enjoy when I hear of young students planning their education journey and working hard to achieve their dreams in life.

Within the Ontario Curriculum the Ministry of Education offers a grade 10 course in career education. In 1999-2000 the Ministry published a new curriculum for Ontario publicly funded schools. Within this new curriculum this grade 10 career education course, which I am qualified to teach, is a phenomenal course as it helps students prepare for life after high school. This open-level course is designed to provide students with the opportunities to discover and develop essential skills for the workplace, college and university. This course is very much hands on, as it allows students to work individually while in group settings, as they take a variety of computer-based quizzes in order to explore what career is best suited for them. While taking this course students will develop their personal management skills in the areas of communication, organization, stress management and conflict resolution. This course also helps students learn about their strengths and weaknesses. I strongly believe that education is an asset for all in order to survive in today's society, and this course helps students begin to think about their future and what they might want to do after they complete high school.

Education is so important for today's youth and I believe the more educated we become the better off we are. As we grow up and begin our careers we may lose jobs and find it hard to seek meaningful employment. However, if we are educated this cannot be taken away from us. I have worked so hard and diligently to obtain my educational dreams, and looking back on it all I do not regret any of my degrees or diplomas.

Teachers' college was such a happy time for me. Everyone was so accommodating to me, and celebrated my successes in life. I was so happy, I had great professors, and one happened to be my high school principal. Carol William was my Human Development professor, and boy was that a fun class. Carol has an awesome personality which made her lectures very enjoyable. There was not one class where I did not find myself laughing out loud from listening to her jokes and fun stories. When I first started teachers college I wasn't 100 per cent sure if I could do it. I was worried about not being able to teach in the final semester. But knowing that Carol was one of my professors encouraged me to continue in the program.

In my final semester of teachers college I applied for a scholarship through the Ontario Federation for Cerebral Palsy to help me pay for my tuition. I needed a few reference letters to include in my application and I had asked Carol to write one for me. I'm not going to share the entire letter, but I will share one part. In her letter she mentioned:

Peter is a very special young man who happens to have cerebral palsy. He does not allow his disability to stop him from participating fully in life. He has powerful skills and level of determination that I have rarely witnessed. Peter has a disability known as Cerebral Palsy. This disability affects the right side of his body as well as his speech. Despite Peter's physical limitations, his cognitive abilities and determination to become a special education teacher and guidance counsellor are truly amazing.

On the most part all of my professors in teachers college were amazing. During the program I took a course in special education where I came across another amazing professor, Dr. Peter Cowden. Dr. Cowden is a retired special education teacher, who is now a university professor at Niagara. I had the privilege of being in two of his courses, special education and assessment. He also taught my sister at her campus. I hate to brag here, but Dr. Cowden `loved` me. He always talked about me in my sister's class, and made me feel like a valued individual. Dr. Cowden's teaching methods were unusual to many. His courses were based on constructive practices. Many teacher candidates were not used to his methods, however, my feeling was that Dr. Cowden taught us `how to teach`. It was a very effective teaching method and one that I used on occasion in my student-teaching practicums.

Attending Niagara University was a very positive and rewarding experience for me. This program is the only teacher training program in Ontario that I know of, which offers teacher candidates exposure to five practice teaching experiences. During the three semesters I taught in four different high schools within York Catholic District School Board. I was placed at St. Brother Andre, St. Therese of Lisieux, St. Maximillian Kolbe and St. Augustine. I chose to stay within the York Catholic board for two reasons: my first reason was because it was easier for me to get to the schools, and secondly I have so many contacts within this board. At the time I felt I was doing the right thing. Having CP makes it challenging for me to drive, therefore I rely on family members and mobility plus, which is a driving program for people with exceptionalities, to get me around town. It was very hard for me to get to other boards like Toronto, Peel and Durham. Therefore, I decided to focus on practice teaching in one school board.

I successfully completed my first year of teachers college, and I had one more semester to go. That summer my parents, sister and myself had planned a family vacation to the States. We had planned on visiting two states, Texas, to visit Kathy, Jim and Nick again, and California. My sister and I had always wanted to visit California for many years, and I had been bugging my mom to take me to Texas since I was young. A highlight of the trip was having the opportunity to go on The Ellen Degeneres Show in Los Angeles. I know most guys don't watch her, but I just love her. On the gloomiest of days all I have to do is watch her on television and my mood changes. We had so much fun on her show, and so many people from Toronto saw us on television. Over the years people have written to Ellen asking her for help in finding a job in the States, however I have not heard back. I would love to work in a special education school in the Deep South, and I have written to Ellen many times in the hopes that she would help me.

We had a great time that summer in California. I love that state. We visited San Diego, Los Angeles, Santa Barbara, Santa Monica, we drove up Big Sir, and ended up in San Francisco, where Kathy's youngest daughter, Kim lives. It was a great trip, and seeing Kim after 20 years was also a highlight of the trip.

I'll never forget, the night before we were about to go home, my mom and dad handed my sister and me a card. Mom said she had forgotten to give it to us on the way to Texas. She gave it to my sister and asked her to read it. When she opened the card it read: "You're Going On A Trip! By train or plan or car or ship…" then my sister opened it and continued reading,

"*Our trip is not over, in fact it's just begun, please share this money between you two for a lot more fun! Let's roll the dice, stay out all night, love each other and promise not to fight.*"

At this point, I knew where we were going. Then the card continued.

"*Can you guess where this will take us, we'll give you a clue… you can't hold on to the cash for more then a minute or two. This place has no clocks, but plenty of lights…Where does this take us….*"

Then my sister turned over the card and on the back it said, "*That's right! Las Vegas!!!!!*" I was so surprised. I've wanted to go there ever since I turned 21. My sister was happy as well, but burst into tears, because she was missing her boyfriend. My mom assured her that it was a short trip, only two nights and one full day. I was a little upset, but didn't say anything. I was thinking who goes to Las Vegas for one day! But I went along with it, and planned out my strategy to see as much of Las Vegas as I possibly could in 24 hours. I knew that sleep was not in my agenda that weekend. We left San Francisco the following afternoon and arrived in Las Vegas that evening. To my sister's surprise and mine, her boyfriend was at the International Airport in Nevada waiting for her. She was so happy, she started crying again. We then found out we were staying there for four days. I was overjoyed; I turned to my mom and said for a joke, "is Nat here?"

Natalie Frances Lind is my long time best friend. We grew up together and met in grade one. Although Nat was not in Vegas that day, we have shared many great times together. Nat is my "Canadian Kathy", as I met her the September following Kathy's big move to Texas. I love her so much. She has always been there for me. She is also a teacher and has been a qualified elementary teacher since 2007. Nat has always been a great friend to me. She has accepted me for who I am, and always defended me whenever I was bullied in elementary school. Nat is my parents "other daughter". She is a kind, compassionate and loyal friend. I am so happy to have her in my life. She is a dedicated and hard working teacher who I absolutely admire.

Well, we came home from our two week trip in the States and an unbelievable four days in Las Vegas. The summer quickly ended and I was back in school; my final semester of teachers college. I had a few courses in August, and I began my practicum teaching in September, on the first day of school. The Niagara University education program in Ontario is very unique, like I mentioned before it is the only program that provides teacher-candidates with five teaching practicums. My first practicum was at my old high school, where I observed a variety of classes and teachers. This observation opportunity allowed me to really examine my host teachers and critique their teaching methods. The one thing I enjoy about teaching is that there is no right way to deliver the curriculum to our students. Teaching is so multi-faceted and as we grow as teachers we learn more about ourselves and what methods best suit our teaching styles. Working with different teachers allows teacher-candidates to learn new styles of teaching. It's very much a "cafeteria-style" of learning. We take what we like about the teachers we worked with, and adapt their methods to develop our own unique method.

Before I had began my practice teaching I foresaw my students as being resilient individuals who would come into my classrooms with open minds and ready to learn. I looked at my classroom as an organization where I was the supervisor and the students were my employees, and education was their primary job in life. After sharing my vision with one of my professors, I soon learned that this vision of mine was idealistic. She told me that as educators we need to have a more realistic vision of our students. It is important for all teachers to understand that at the core of all students lay vulnerable individuals who come into our classrooms from all walks of life. Through my educational training and practice teaching, I have learned that teachers are given enormous responsibilities besides the deliverance of the curriculum. Many people mock teachers for having three months off each year and a job that allows them to work for nine in the morning to three-thirty in the afternoon, but this is not true. Teachers are constantly working around the clock, preparing for daily their lesson plans and making sure that they are properly teaching students each year. Reality is that we are not just teachers. We are daytime parents, lawyers who help students resolve conflict, nurses who heals all sorts of wounds, we are therapists who help students deal with all kinds of problems and with all that we deal with, we manage to be teachers, who are focused on our careers and help students succeed through their own academic journey's and strive to see them reach their full potential.

In my first teaching practicum in the final semester of teachers college, I was placed at St. Brother Andre C.H.S., where I worked with two teachers, Mary Ronan and Ted Titus. These two teachers praised the ground I walked on. I was constantly told by them what a great job I was doing. I was supposed to do my two placements, teaching religion and geography, at two different schools, but after teaching in Mary's religion classes, I had a hard time finding a second placement so I worked with Ted in his geography class. I had the opportunity to work with a geography teacher at Sutton District High School, but unfortunately I passed up this opportunity because the school was too far for me to get to five days a week. I was enjoying my time at St. Brother Andre C.H.S, so I decided to stay. The school's principal at the time, Mr. Jim Nicoletti got wind of how well I was teaching and observed me teaching in Mary's class. He was impressed with my methods, and that semester before he retired he offered to mock interview me. I was a bit nervous; it was my first interview with a principal. It didn't go as well as I hoped, however, Mr. Nicoletti said he appreciated my responses, but informed me that I needed to focus more on what the Board was looking for in my answers.

I was very fortunate to have the opportunity to do my placements in my old high school. I was very nervous beginning my teaching semester as I wasn't sure how well students were going to respond to me. I am first to admit that my voice is not that clear, and the volume is not always loud enough. I did struggle in the beginning; however, Mary eased me into teaching. I taught two of her classes on a full time basis, and her third class periodically. The university that I was attending was actively looking for a portable microphone that I could use in my classroom. However, in the meantime my students were very understanding of my limitations, and instead of mocking me, they paid extra attention to my lessons.

Once Niagara University found a suitable microphone for me, I was very successful. This device was a portable unit that had a speaker and wireless microphone. I placed the speaker in a corner of the classroom and I had the microphone clipped on my shirt. If my students didn't hear me, I would simply ask them to increase the volume on the speaker. Each day that I came into school I always entered with a smile, and left with a smile. I was in my glory. Students were respecting me both within the school and the community. My last name, Mitskinis, is very hard to pronounce for the average person, so I always got called "Sir" or "Mr. M". I felt like an important person. I never felt like this in my life.

When I finished both my placements with Mary and Ted, they wrote me amazing evaluations and outstanding reference letters. One of my star students, a grade 10 by the name of Taylor Cannon, was asked by Mary if he to would write me a letter of reference. He was delighted to do this for me. At the time Taylor was 14 years old, and I remember sitting at my desk while he was typing the letter all by himself. After he was finished I could not believe the vocabulary that this kid had. I need to share with you what he wrote:

Re: Mr. Mitskinis

To Whom It May Concern:
As a student of Mr. Mitskinis` I must commend him on his fantastic performance as both a class teacher and a mentor. His effective and engaging class activities encouraged both me and my peers to delve deep into ourselves in order to resolve both personal and moral questions relating to the program and our lives. Mr. Mitskinis did an outstanding job of organizing both class discussions and individual study periods in order to further our understanding of the themes. His absolute devotion to the success of his students and his exceptional teaching techniques display his effectiveness in an instructing position and I believe he will make a phenomenal teacher. It was a pleasure to be in his class and I look forward to any opportunities I have to be taught by him in the future.

Sincerely, Taylor Cannon

When I read this I was flabbergasted. I was so impressed; I came home that night and showed my parents. My mom read it and cried. I attended parent-teacher night that semester with my host teachers where I had the privilege of meeting Ms. Cannon, Taylor's mom. I told her what an awesome son she had, and that night when I came home I wrote her a letter thanking her for raising such a wonderful son. I also attached Taylor's letter to my letter so that she could see it as well. Apparently, Taylor told me it made her day, and she was so happy. I never met Taylor's father, but I know for a fact, if I were his dad, I would be so proud of my son.

During my placements, I taught grade 9 and 10 religion as well as grade 9 geography. The semester was moving along and my field placement supervisor, Frank Fazzari, came to watch me teach for the third time. We had four scheduled visits all together, two for each placement. During this visit Frank was a little worried that I was getting too comfortable at St. Brother Andre, and suggested I try a different school. He told me that this would help me get to know other principals and experience a different school atmosphere. I finished off teaching my geography unit in Ted's class, and went to a new school (St. Augustine's) where I met George Lambrosopoulous. Fortunately this school was in Markham, and not too far away from where I live.

St. Augustine is a great school. The principal, Bernie Smith, was very welcoming, and I found out that we attended Mass at the same Parish. I enjoyed my time there as well. The students were very bright, a little bit shy and quiet, but so much fun to work with. George was a terrific host teacher and he enjoyed watching me teach. When my supervisor came to observe me at this school, he was very impressed. This high school was a perfect fit for me. It is a very high tech school and they offer students a laptop program. This allows students to work on their own laptop while the teacher conducted their lessons on a Smartboard. Like my other placements, I used power point software to conduct my daily lessons. Also because I have a speech impairment I used a wireless voice enhancer that the university finally found for me to help me increase my volume level. The one thing I like about being a teacher is that in a way you become the manager of your own classroom. This allows teachers to make their classroom a welcoming environment that is adaptable to both their own needs as well as the needs of their students. I successfully completed my practicums, and all that was left to do was to look forward to our graduation.

My students in both placements were surprisingly amazing. A few times during the semester my peers would meet up at the university to discuss how our placements were going. I could not believe some of the stories that I heard my peers tell about their students. I was so fortunate with my students at St. Brother Andre CHS and St. Augustine CHS. For the most part my students were attentive, well mannered, and fascinated with my teaching methods. They seemed so happy to be in my class. I was firm yet made learning fun. I only had one student call me "mean", and that was only because there are two things that I do not tolerate in class, and these are, no talking when someone else or myself is talking, and no cell phones or electronic devices during class. I remember this student was using her phone in class, and after telling her more then once to put it away, I confiscated it and placed it on my desk. Later that day she came back to get her cell phone and I explained how distracting cell phones can be in class. She was apologetic and I returned her phone.

Being firm with students doesn't mean that you are a mean teacher; it simply means that you are there to teach them and it is their job to learn. Mutual respect in any school environment is a two-way street. It is built on respect and when teachers show respect to their students, then they are more inclined to receive it back.

Many of the teacher candidates at Niagara University had horror stories about some of the students they were teaching and the schools they were teaching at. I was so impressed and lucky with how much my students respected me and listened to me. Now don't get me wrong, they weren't always "little angels" everyday; they had their moments when they would act inappropriately in class and drive me bananas. However, overall they were so respectful and enjoyed my classes. Whenever they see me volunteering in their schools, or within the community, they always say "hi sir" and ask me how I am doing. In my reference letter from Mary Ronan, she mentioned how well students were responding to me. Her exact words were, "their acceptance quickly escalated to respect and admiration for Peter's teaching abilities as well as his goodness which is readily apparent on a daily and consistent basis."

When teaching with Mary we had an awesome relationship, and we still do to this very day. Mary really helped me develop as a teacher and she always made me feel good about myself. Working with Mary made my practicum experience go extremely well. Not one day was I overly stressed. I did have my moments, but Mary always seemed to make the small problems insignificant. The one thing I learned about Mary and her teaching style was that students really enjoyed her class. She made learning enjoyable and her classroom is a place where everyone is equal. Equality in a classroom is so important, and I learned this so well from her.

She made me realize that students come into our classrooms each day with all sorts of baggage, besides their backpack and gym bag. Many students often come to school with empty stomachs, problems at home, drug problems, health issues and in many cases there are student who deal with separated or divorced parents. There were many times when Mary could tell that students came to class starving, even after their lunch period. Many times she would offer them a few bucks to go and purchase some food from the school's cafeteria. This act of kindness was so exhilarating for me to see; and I know that I would do the same for my students when I begin teaching. Students should be able to talk to their teachers and ask them for help when needed. Teachers can easily direct students to help within the school community if they cannot find help for themselves. At the high school level, students have access to guidance counsellors, vice-principals, principals, coaches, mentors, a number of teachers, and in the Catholic high schools they offer chaplains. My goal is to also be a chaplain one day. These teachers have an important role in Catholic schools. The organize retreats for students, school Masses and liturgies, and provide spiritual counselling to students. I believe that chaplaincy would be another terrific area for me to work in as an educator.

Well, my final semester in teachers college was a huge success. My sister and I finished our program in December of 2010, and graduation was scheduled for January. My family had a wonderful Christmas that year, and we were able to go down south after New Years to enjoy our new condo for the first time. It was an awesome way to end a very busy semester. We had a wonderful time in Florida, and we enjoyed using our condo. My family and I have been going to Florida almost every year since I was a baby. It is like our second home. My grandparents have their own house and business down there, and they too enjoy spending the winters in Florida. Unfortunately our trip got cut short. Prior to Christmas my grandmother was on the list for bypass surgery and got called to come in on January 21st, 2011. I was so worried for her, so we all came home to support her. The one thing about my family (especially mom's side), we are very supportive of each other.

The operation was scheduled for the day after we arrived home. I really wanted to go and sit in the waiting room so badly, but my grandmother told me not to. If there were ever a day in my life that I prayed the hardest that was it. The operation was three hours long, but it felt like eternity. That day I received so many calls from family and friends asking about grandma's status. Fortunately, everything went well and grandma has fully recovered and is enjoying going back and forth to Florida. Unfortunately she missed my sister and my graduation ceremony, however, Aunt Josie and my cousin Antonella came in our grandparents place. I also invited my friend Terri Penney to watch us graduate.

LIFE AFTER TEACHERS COLLEGE

Since graduating from teachers college in December 2010 I have been busy. I have taken two additional qualification courses in special education and guidance. OECTA, which is the Ontario Education Catholic Teachers Association, gave me equivalency for religion part 1 and 2, because of my undergraduate degree in religious studies. All Catholic education teachers are required to have at least part 1. I am so grateful that I was granted these courses, because taking additional qualification courses can be costly. Now I am officially qualified to teach religious studies, geography, special education and guidance and career education. I have everything I need to teach, except for a job. I was interviewed on April 1st, 2011 (and no this was not an April Fools joke), for the York Catholic school board as an occasional teacher. The interview was at St. Brother Andre C.H.S., and I was interviewed by the principal and one of the vice principals. I was so nervous. My sister and I had been preparing each other for our interviews. We asked each other questions, reflected on what we had learned in teachers college, and what we had learned during each of our placements.

The faculty at my teaching program had set up mock interviews for all teacher candidates before our graduation. Principals from different school boards had come to the university to mock interview all of the teacher candidates. This was very beneficial for me as it helped me feel what a Board interview would be like, although you never know what kinds of questions you will be asked in the real interview. Looking back I believe that it is important for all teacher-candidates to be truthful in an interview and highlight your strengths and what you can bring forth to your classroom.

The one thing about being interviewed for a school board is that they look for specific key ideas and terms in you responses. I remember sweating so much during the interview. Prior to my interview people told me to just take my time and answer the questions the best I could, but that is easier said then done.

Towards the end of the school year I took another trip to Texas, but this time I went on my own to celebrate my birthday with Kathy and her family. It was great too see them all again. I had the time of my life. When I returned home, the high school students were about to begin exams, therefore, there was no need for me to go in and volunteer. Summer began and my family took another trip to Florida with my mom's cousins. We had a great time. Steph had found out that she was hired as a substitute teacher for Toronto Catholic District School Board, and I was patiently waiting to hear from York Catholic District School Board. Unfortunately on August 17th, I received the news. I was told that in relation to the Boards current staffing needs, at this time they were unable to offer me a position. I was so disappointed. All that hard work and dedication, and now I find out I didn't even get hired. However the e-mail did mention that,

"Your employment application will remain active for a two year school period. It is recommended that you continue to update your on-line application with any relevant information

such as additional qualifications, practice teaching reports, teacher evaluations or letters of reference.”

Although I was so upset and devastated, I have been doing exactly what they said. I have been updating my profile with the Board. I added my special education and guidance and career education qualification courses, and received a few reference letters to add to my online file.

Since then I have also looked into alternative means of employment. To this day I have applied to many different positions, twenty-four of which have to do with education in some form. These include, private schools, tutoring companies and I also applied to different Boards for different teaching positions. I have been overwhelmed and stressed. Nobody is hiring these days. I understand that there are people who have applied to hundreds of positions and nothing has come up. However, because of my physical limitations, many of the jobs out there do not apply to me. I could never work in areas like construction, retail, and restaurants because of my physical limitations.

It is tough living in today’s world when you have a disability. Non-disabled people will never know the feeling of what it is like to see the world from my perspective. I am not saying this so that you can feel sorry for me, my intention is to make others aware of what many educated people with exceptionalities are facing each and every day of their lives. Can you imagine working hard on your career goals and then once you have all the education and necessary experiences, there is no job for you. It is devastating to many, especially me. I try so hard to put on a happy face and my parents constantly remind me, that there are others who are worse off then me.

My personal beliefs as a teacher

After studying education and pursuing employment opportunities, I have learned that a passionate teacher is faithful at his core, to his beliefs, his values, his ideas, and works to share these with those God has gifted him to teach. Teaching is a privilege; not just a job. To help in the formation of a young person is an awesome responsibility, and I cannot wait until I am given this opportunity. As a newly educated teacher perhaps I am idealistic and I know experience in the classroom will make me more realistic in time. However, I hope and pray that I will be a witness to what is best in my life, to the things that really matter, and whether the students I teach ever remember anything I say, he or she will remember that I treated him or her with respect and that I truly cared about each and every student of mine. My fears as a teacher are that I will not be able to reach everyone at the level I would like. But I understand that the meaning of the word "teach" is to "lead forth", so that is what I aim to do-to lead others to become all they can be. Students will be entrusted to me for a certain period of time, and perhaps the best I can do is plant seeds for further growth. The work is not mine alone and the work is not about me. I see teaching as being of service to others, of making myself available to others, and that is certainly a Gospel principle which Jesus the great Teacher showed me. Especially as a prospective religious education, special education teacher and guidance counsellor, I hope to lead by example by being myself. I know I have limitations as does each and every person. We are all vulnerable and sometimes wounded, and that's all right, because it will be my humanity as well as the grace of God which will shine through.

Deep down I feel that God is personally calling me to pursue a profession in teaching. As I have mentioned before, I began my post-secondary education journey in college studying Journalism-Print, however when it came to participate in my field placement portion of this program, it was then that I realized that this career was not for me. The journalism profession is an ongoing job that I found extremely fast-paced. Although I completed my college diploma at Durham College, I just wasn't ready for this type of career. Despite my physical limitations, I sense God has been directing me through my journey and leading me to a career as a teacher. I believe that He wants me to enter into this career so that I can continue to be a role model for future students. I believe that it is important for me to take teaching seriously, because it is my passion, my goal and above all it is definitely my calling in life. There are many aspects of teaching that are important for me. I want to continue learning all that I can about the role of the special education teacher and guidance counsellor, as I feel that these areas will make me a more marketable teacher. I can honestly say that I would make a terrific addition in either of these specialty areas. But above all, I think that realizing not only who I am, but whose I am, namely God's, will enable me to let this inner teacher/spirituality shine through.

Right now my volunteer experience in elementary and secondary schools within the York Catholic District School Board has me working in the special education department with children of all ages and abilities. This is such a rich experience for me. Working with students who have exceptionalities is both a complex and rewarding job. The job of a special education teacher is very different from the regular classroom teacher. The special education teacher plays an important role in the successful inclusion of students with exceptionalities. Everyday is different in special education departments across the country, and it is important for educators to adapt to different challenges and learn as we go along. I believe that teachers need to give 100 per cent of their time, talents and treasures in order to truly become a successful teacher.

For me, success is not determined by the number of degrees that hang on your wall, I believe that success is measured by the obstacles we overcome and how we deal with challenges in life. I am still dealing with personal challenges of my own, but I try to stay positive, remain focused on my dreams and continue on in life as God would want me to. So many times I have often wondered what my purpose in life is. I have been actively searching for employment in other sectors since all school boards are currently over-staffed, however, when it comes down to the nitty-gritty of what I want to do with life, I am constantly being directed to teaching. Is it my own imagination? I can honestly say it's not. I believe God is molding me, guiding me and using me as a prospective teacher.

STANDARDS OF PRACTICE FOR THE TEACHING PROFESSION

As I have mentioned before, my ultimate goal as a teacher is to work in the areas of special education, guidance and career education as well as chaplaincy. These areas are ideal for me and my abilities as an educator. I feel that working one-on-one would be a great job for me. After learning about education as a profession, one of the most important aspects to this job is the Standards of Practice for the Teaching Profession. As an aspiring teacher, I have learned a great deal about these standards. These five standards are important for all teachers to adhere to as they provide them with a theoretical framework for teaching students in Ontario. They describe the knowledge, skills and values that are necessary for the teaching profession. These standards convey collective vision of professionalism that guides a daily practice of teachers. As a prospective special education teacher and guidance councillor these standards can effectively help me as I work with students, and assist them with any challenge that he or she is facing. Unlike other professions, teachers are fortunate to have these standards as they identify the values, knowledge and skills that are important to obtain as teachers. They help guide professional judgement and promote a common language that assists teachers to understand what it means to be an effective teacher.

Teaching is a profession that calls professionals to work in collaboration with their colleagues in order to improve the delivery of the curriculum to our students. The standards of practice for the teaching profession are important for teachers to take into consideration as they are meant to inspire a shared vision for all teachers and identify the values, knowledge and skills that are distinctive. The standards are also there to help guide professional judgement and daily actions. Lastly, they promote a common language that fosters an understanding of what it means to be a valuable member of the teaching profession. The first standard is known as Commitment to Students and Student Learning.

The most important aspect of teaching is to work in a collaborative fashion as this allows teachers to dedicate themselves to their vocation and to their students. Being committed to teaching and students is extremely imperative for educators to do. It is crucial for teachers to care for students equitably and with respect, while being sensitive to the factors that influences their learning. Showing that you are interested in the learning process of students allows teachers to treat their students like important individuals who are valuable contributors to our Canadian society. By being committed to our students and their learning, will help them develop their skills and strive for excellence as they continue on their education paths.

In order to effectively teach any academic or applied level subjects, teachers must recognize the importance of professional knowledge. The second standards, which is the practice of professional knowledge is vital for teachers to adhere to. As a teacher I know how important it is to stay current in this profession and constantly reflect on their students' development, learning theory, pedagogy, curriculum, ethics, and education research. Teachers also need to be in touch with educational policies and legislation in order to improve professional judgement throughout their profession. One way teachers can advance their professional knowledge is through constantly educating themselves. This can be done by taking additional qualification courses, attending professional workshops/seminars, and keeping themselves up to date with knowledge of educational practices and issues within their community. With their professional knowledge teachers can effectively apply it to their practice and promote student learning. In order to perfect their practice, teachers need to use appropriate pedagogy, assessment and evaluation strategies, as well as resources, technology and tactics that will effectively help them plan, respond to the needs of their students and enhance the learning environment.As teachers it is also important to remember that we are all leaders within our school communities. It is imperative that we work together with our colleagues to make our schools a collaborative, safe and supportive learning community for all members. In order to facilitate student success teachers must recognize their shared responsibilities as well as their leadership roles that will help them be a part of their student's achievement. Since we are called to be professionals, we must maintain and uphold the principles of ethical standards when working within our learning communities as we are constantly role models for our students. Lastly, the final standard teaches educators that teaching is a profession that involves ongoing learning on their part. It is important for teachers to frequently educate themselves in order to effectively teach their students and keep up with the changes in education to help their students succeed. When teachers exercise these five standards it allows them to become actively involved in practicing and improving their teaching methods and strategies. Teaching is an important profession that should be entered into with deep dedication and commitment. When teachers absolutely love what they do, this encourages them to improve their skills and become better teachers to educate and improve the future of their students.

The field of education is forever changing, and in order to keep up with its demands, teachers need to commit themselves to ongoing professional learning. This type of self-directed learning allows teachers to continue learning through taking additional qualification courses, attending teaching-related workshops and seminars, increasing the use of technology in their classrooms and keeping up with educational practices through reading educational-related journals and other resources. As a guidance counsellor it is important to keep up with new practices that will help you better counsel your students. Right now I have graduated at a time where it is tough to obtain a teaching position in Ontario; therefore, instead of doing nothing and just waiting for a job, I have taken additional qualification courses to help me learn more about the areas in education that I hope to work in, namely special education and guidance. I am also volunteering in local schools to keep practicing and learning new teaching methods.

Lastly, in order to maintain professionalism in teaching, it is important that teachers apply their professional knowledge to their teaching. When teachers constantly practice their teaching techniques this helps them perform better each day. It is important for teachers to refine their professional practice by using appropriate pedagogy, different types of assessment and evaluation methods, and a variety of resources and technology in their lesson planning. Although I am unemployed, I found myself using a variety of different teaching methods during my practicums in teachers college and now when I volunteer in local schools. It is important for teachers to make learning both fun and educational for students. When a teacher effectively grabs their student's attention and successfully hooks them into a lesson, then this helps the learning process become successful. Upon further review of the policy documents from the Ministry of Education, I find their directions are similarly stated as with the Standards of Practice for the Teaching Profession.

TEACHERS ALSO NEED TO KNOW THE ETHICAL STANDARDS FOR THE TEACHING PROFESSION

The Ethical Standards for the Teaching Profession is another document for teachers. This document represents a vision of professional practice. For me, it is the combination of my experiences from high school, teachers college and practice teaching. I have learned how committed my teachers were to me to see that I always progressed forward. As I went through teachers college and practice teaching, I also felt the responsibility and relationship with my students to do the best I could, to teach them and to move forward. I also realized the importance of my connections with my colleagues at the schools to learn from them as much as possible, and make use of any other professional in the school system. By working with colleagues, this will help me with my goal of educating my students. The purposes of the ethical standards are to inspire teachers to reflect and uphold the honour and dignity of the teaching profession. There are four ethical standards, care, respect, trust and integrity. As teachers it is important for us to show that we are compassionate towards our students and be accepting and respectful of each and every student we teach as well as the colleagues we work with. It is important for teachers, especially guidance counsellors to show that they care for their student's well-being and learning process. During my practice teaching it was important for me to show that I care for my students by answering their questions and making myself available to help them before or after school. I was able to assist those who were struggling, I was compassionate towards those who needed accommodations, and shared their interests and related them to the course material. When students know that their teachers care about them and their education, then this creates a positive atmosphere for everyone and encourages them to do well in school. This makes it easier for students to trust in their teachers abilities and respect them for all the work that they put into the teaching profession.

As a prospective guidance counsellor and special education teacher, I feel it is also important to get a sense of the different family systems within out school communities. By getting to know the parents of our students, then this will help us understand where our students come from. In situations where we suspect a hostile living environment where students might be experiencing abuse, negligence, etc, then I feel that it is important for guidance counsellor's to step in and try to help the student overcome their troubles at home. It is important to set up guidance appointments with these students and let them know that you are there to help them in anyway possible. You want the student to feel comfortable and you want to develop a trust with the student and only then will they come and talk to you openly about their problems. If students come to us saying that their parents abuse them, then I believe that it is our duty and the law to report the situation to Child Services, and follow-up with them. I do not believe that we, guidance counsellors, have the right to confront parents ourselves.

However, if we deal with situations in a professional manner, then it becomes easier to help our students rectify all kinds of family issues. I do not feel that the age of the student should influence whether or not a guidance counsellor should step in and help. If we are told by a student that there are family problems at home, or we suspect that a student is having problems, then I feel it is our moral and civil duty to help them as much as we can.

WHY IT IS IMPORTANT FOR ME TO BE A CATHOLIC TEACHER

My experiences that I have been sharing with you have taught me that teaching is a vocation that calls the best of the best to educate today's youth for tomorrow's future. As a teacher who has experience teaching in Catholic schools, it is important for me to model my teaching techniques after our Lord and Saviour, Jesus Christ. My goal is as a guidance counsellor, school chaplain and special educator, is to work one-on-one with students, to help them overcome any type of challenge they may experience in life. As a Catholic, my faith is extremely important to me, and as an educator I hope to bring both Catholic and moral values into my classroom environment to better the learning environment. By pursuing my dreams of becoming a Catholic educator I stand for many values and beliefs, which I hope to, bring into my classroom and instil into my students.

There are many Catholic values that I, as a teacher, would like my students to model while in my class. I look forward to making my classroom an environment that is built on the core values of faith, hope, love, and compassion with the focus on mutual respect for one another. These values, when put in place, can give school communities the opportunity to clearly express their faith as they live out these values in their daily lives. As a teacher I plan on incorporating these core values into my classroom as well as into my lesson plans, by modeling them myself. I plan to start off each academic year, by setting the tone and expectations of both my students and myself and work hard towards meeting them. Since I plan on teaching in the Catholic school system, I will focus on faith beliefs as the moral compass of how my classroom will flow. Having faith in our Saviour, Jesus Christ is important to me, and I would hope my students would respect those who have a strong faith in God. If students begin to see me as a compassionate, spiritual and dedicated teacher, who respects everyone for who they are, then hopefully, my students will see me as a role model, and learn to practice what I preach (or teach).

As the years move on in my teaching career, I hope to leave behind a positive legacy for my students, one that they will remember, that even though our time together has come to an end, I will always be in their school community for any guidance and support they may need. Once students move on and experience new teachers, I would want them to remember me as a fun, motivated, and outgoing teacher who enjoys the challenge that teaching brings, as well as an individual who makes learning experiences both enjoyable and educational at the same time. I would also want my students to look at me and see that with hard work, perseverance, dedication and determination anything in life is possible, as long as you put your mind toward pursuing your dreams. It is also important for me to make sure that students know that having a strong faith in God can help us conquer any of life's obstacles.

WHAT I FEEL IS IMPORTANT IN TODAY'S EDUCATION SYSTEM!

In a profession like education it is important for teachers to make long-term goals for themselves. As an educator I have many ideas and long-term goals that I plan on fulfilling once I am employed by an Ontario school board. Since the days when my parents attended school, education has come a long way. The biggest evolution in education, and perhaps the most significant one, is the inclusion of students with special needs. According to one of my special needs textbooks, entitled, *Teaching Students with Special Needs in Inclusive Settings* by Tom E.C. Smith et al., the authors mention that in Canada, the movement towards inclusion was somewhat slower. When reading this textbook one comment stood out to me; they said, "normalization proponents believed that all individuals, regardless of disability, should be provided with an education and a living arrangement as normal as possible" (Smith et al., 2006, 3). As a teacher I want to help the education system come up with new innovations that will benefit the student with an exceptionality and enable them to become a valuable individual in the classroom as well as within their school community.

As teachers, I believe it is important to celebrate students' achievements and abilities, and work with what a student can do. When working in special education, it is important for teachers to collaborate with the special education teacher as well as the student, to make sure his or her needs are being met in the classroom throughout each school year. I also believe that teachers need to be advocates for students with exceptionalities. We live in a society that is not always accommodating to those with exceptionalities; therefore, educators must make it their moral obligation to help these students become all they can be.

When teachers have students with exceptionalities in their classroom, I believe that we need to help them find their skills and highlight their abilities. For all we know the next student with an exceptionality that we teach could in fact be the next humanitarian who makes a difference in society. I would like to see our education system become even more evolved and help celebrate students with exceptionalities and their uniqueness.

According to the Education Act on Special Education, this document states that it is: "the responsibility of school boards to provide (or to purchase from another board) special education programs and special education services for their exceptional pupils" (paragraph 7 of subsection 170(1). My parish, St. Patrick's, has a slogan that they use to represent the parish vision, and I strongly feel that it is so fitting in education. This slogan goes like this: "To Be Faithful Servants Walking God's Talk." Those working in the field of education need to be accepting of everyone; as we are all crafted in God's image and likeness. God doesn't judge us on our abilities, or lack there of. He does however judge us on what we did or didn't do for others, and how we made a difference in their lives. When we see students with exceptionalities participating in mainstream education, it is important for teachers to be accommodating of their needs and help them achieve academic success. Just like the Great Teacher, we need to treat others with kindness and respect in ways that Jesus did 2000 years ago.

Nowadays, Canadian public schools show greater compassion for children with exceptionalities than they did in the past. I once read a book by Charles Undergerleider entitled *Failing Our Kids*, and he had some interesting outlooks on teaching students with exceptionalities. The most significant idea that he mentioned in his book was, "the end results of education for most special-needs children should be no different from the results we are trying to achieve for all students," (Undergerleider, 2003, 127). Why should teachers treat these students any differently than their non-disabled peers? In many cases children with exceptionalities will achieve more if their needs are properly identified in their early years. My goal as a special education teacher is to really examine each student that I work with, and properly pinpoint their strengths and needs. If teachers do too much for students, then this becomes problematic as they will become too dependent on their support. The same goes for the opposite situation, if teachers do not provide students with enough support, then they will be pushed through the education system and will suffer in the end.

Working with children who have exceptionalities is a lot like baking a cake. If we add to many ingredients to the mix, the cake will not turn out, whereas if there are not enough, then we need to keep working on it until it turns out the way we like it. Now, it is important to remember that when we work in a special education department, we as teachers need to listen to our students and understand their needs and what they want help with. If we do to much or not enough for our students, then we are doing them no favours in life.

WHAT I HAVE LEARNED WHILE I AM WAITING FOR A JOB!

While I have been volunteering in schools like St. Brother Andre's special education department as well at All Saints Catholic School which is an elementary school in Markham, I am learning more about special education, and I am gaining more practical experience. I have been working with a wide-range of students of different ages and exceptionalities. I am very grateful that both schools have given me this opportunity to volunteer as I am really enjoying myself. Working in special education is such a rewarding yet challenging profession. Over the years I have gained experience working with students who have cerebral palsy (like me), autism spectrum disorder, spina bifida, Downs syndrome, as well as learning disabilities. Each student is so unique and I have learned a great deal from each of them.

When working with students who have exceptionalities, it makes me feel really good about myself when I know that my assistance and dedication has helped them better develop their skills. I have learned through my experiences in special education that each student is different and we need to work with them and help them develop their skills. The Charter of Rights and Freedoms, states that Canada has become the first country in the world to protect the rights of people with disabilities in a constitution. According to section 15 (1) it says that,

Every individual is equal before and under the law and has the right to equal protection of the law without discrimination based on race, nationality or ethnic origin, colour, religion, sex, age, or mental or physical disability.

Therefore it is our duty as educators to promote education for all, and integrate those with exceptionalities into the mainstream classroom as much as possible. Every school board in Ontario has a duty and responsibility to provide special education programs and services to exceptional pupils. According to section 1 of the *Education Act* they define "exceptional pupil" is "a pupil whose behaviour, communicational, intellectual, physical, or multiple exceptionalities are such that he or she is considered to need placement in a special education program [an Identification, Placement and Review Committee] of the board," (Ontario Education Act on Special Education, Subsection 1(1)).

I am very blessed because despite my physical limitations, students respond to me and my teaching methods very well. Whenever I volunteer in schools students are constantly thanking me for helping them and asking me if I will be coming back the following day. When I tell them I will be in, their faces light up and I know that I have made an impact in their lives. Students with exceptionalities are like anyone else, they have feelings; many know and understand what they want and enjoy being a part of any community. Although many students cannot express their emotions, I have learned that we all need to be patient with them and reinforce positive behaviour and skills, and help them become valued students within their school.

When teaching children of any age, gender, race, ability etc, we have to keep in mind what God says about humanity. In the book of Genesis, which is the first book of the Old Testament, as well as the first book of the Bible, we read: "so God created human beings in his own image. In the image of God he created them; male and female he created them," (Genesis 1:27). I believe that this means that God has a purpose for each and every person on this Earth. There are times when I have trouble seeing what my purpose in life is; then there are times when God reminds me of my purpose in life whenever I successfully help a student. Whether it's in a classroom helping a student complete a task that they had been struggling with, or during my RCIA meetings when non-baptized people ask me questions about our faith or even helping a friend out in times of need. In many ways I truly believe that God is guiding me to make good use of my time, talents and treasures.

In life there are times when we find it challenging to accept people for who they are and what they have done to us. I know that there have been people who have disappointed me, and I have been taught that we need to look for Jesus in everyone we meet. This is especially important for teachers to consider. In a profession like teaching, emotions can run wild among teachers. I have learned that teachers need to control their emotions in order to be successful at their job.

When individuals first begin a career in teaching, many immediately grasp the art of teaching and their inner teacher-spirit shines right through them. This makes it easy for others to tell that these teachers really enjoy what they do. Their job becomes so natural for them, and it is easy to tell that these teachers enjoy their profession. There is an old saying that states: "choose a job you love and you will never have to work a day in your life." I truly believe this, because whenever I have volunteered in various classrooms, I have really enjoyed the interaction with the students, and I have taken great pleasure in helping the students complete their work. Teaching feels so natural to me, that it doesn't feel like I'm working when in the classroom.

I strongly feel that natural teachers are the ones who make a welcoming classroom environment. These individuals are confident with their performance, and show interest in their students and the work they do. Natural teachers are individuals who bring energy and confidence to their classroom. The teaching profession is very spontaneous; teachers should learn to expect all kinds of students and situations that they must deal with. In any situation, natural teachers are the ones who make effective teaching creative. Therefore, teachers need to be open-minded and must expect distraction in their classroom.

New teachers must realize that students often take advantage of them. In these situations I believe teachers must not let students control them, but rather manage their students and classroom in order to maintain a positive learning atmosphere. I was told that when someone begins their teaching career, if they survive their first five years then they will have a successful future in teaching. I believe that natural teachers have great abilities to accept any situation in the classroom and deal with it in the most appropriate manner.

Another key quality that natural teachers possess is knowing about teaching and the learning process. I believe it is important for teachers to learn as much as they can about their profession. The best thing a teacher can do is invest in themselves. We have limitless opportunities to learn knew teaching methods through additional qualification courses as well as participating in teaching seminars and workshops. The more qualified a teacher becomes, the more they can offer to their students and perfect their art of teaching. When teachers keep themselves abreast of new teaching methods this has a huge impact on their performance, as they become an expert in their subject area. I believe natural teachers are confident in the way they plan and deliver a lesson.

Like any profession, being a natural teacher involves a great deal of preparation; it also involves continual practice and reflection over time. I believe we need to be reflective teachers so that we can see where we went wrong in a lesson, and look for ways to improve. Through constant practice and reflection, I really believe that this helps all teachers improve their skills and make appropriate changes in future lessons.

At the beginning of each academic year, or semester, I feel that natural teachers need to set a tone for his or her class, and lay out their classroom expectations. In order to make learning enjoyable these teachers need to be creative and make wise decisions that relate to teaching and the learning process. In my past teaching experiences, I feel that when students are aware of my (the teacher's) expectations and are engaged in the lessons, they tend to be better behaved and enjoy the classroom experience immensely. There are so many natural teachers out there, and I hope to one day be one of them. I want to help encourage my students to be the best that they can in life, and learn from my experiences since I was once a student just like them. I think that it is important for teachers to feel comfortable with their students as this will allow for better communication and a successful academic year. Being confident in what you do is essential for a successful natural teacher. There is a song by the famous singer, Whitney Houston about children, and one of her lyrics says,

"I believe the children are our future, teach them well and let them lead the way, show them all the beauty they possess inside, give them a sense of pride to make it easier. Let the children's laughter remind us how we used to be!"

These lyrics are so fitting for every teacher to live by, and consider when working in the classroom.

As the years move on and education continues to change, I believe that general education teachers will be seeing more and more students with exceptionalities being integrated in their classroom. I would love to be a part of this process and see this change come to fruition. I believe it's important to get non-disabled students involved in this change. I see how much of an asset peers can be for these students, and together they can learn from each other. There are many students with hidden exceptionalities that teachers need to watch out for in their classroom. When teachers suspect a student has some kind of exceptionality then they need to get in touch with the special education teacher. This teacher will see if the student has been identified, and what accommodations and modifications he or she requires to be academically successful.

When it comes to assisting students with exceptionalities, it is important for special education teachers to know the difference between accommodations and modifications, as these two terms greatly differ from one another. While analyzing students IEPs teachers need to become aware of different aspects of the curriculum that needs to be modified, and then implement the accommodations to help the student with their courses. Accommodations are supports or services that are not provided to the general student population, however they are required by individual students with special needs to help them achieve learning expectations and demonstrate learning. Whereas modifications are changes in the curriculum to help the student academically succeed.

Teaching students with exceptionalities can be a tricky job. It is important to provide supports that are suitable to their needs. Accommodations are referred to as specialized supports and services provide to enable students with exceptionalities to participate in their everyday learning environments. When providing students with accommodations, these can range from technological equipment, support staff, and informal supports. Accommodations are different from modifications because they are more of a support service that the student will use to reach the goals of the curriculum. As I mentioned above accommodations are changing how the student learns. For example, providing the students with a computer or note taker to help them with their writing is an example of an accommodation that some students may need. During my practice teaching experiences I have had to incorporate accommodations into my lesson plans as I had a student with a learning disability (LD) in one of my classes. One of the most common accommodations that students with LD needs is breaking up work and giving students extra time to complete their work. Student with LD may feel overwhelmed and tend to work on assignments better when given in small increments. When working with students who have exceptionalities it is important to know that no single method always works. Teachers need to individualize their efforts when accommodating students, as no student is the same.

As mentioned above, modifications are changes to the curriculum that will support students with exceptionalities in their learning. When teachers are developing modified expectations, they need to make important decisions regarding the skills and knowledge that need to be taught. A modification is simply a change from the expected outcome. In my teaching experiences I have had to provide modifications for the same student that I mentioned above, by making the curriculum a bit more manageable by reducing the workload. This can be done by having the student focus on less material then the rest of the class. When making modifications for students, these changes must be both age and grade-appropriate, for a subject or course. If a student does not understand what he or she is being taught, the teacher must change (modify) the curriculum to make it more manageable for the student in order to learn effectively. Lastly, modifications are made when the accommodations in the IEP are not working. Therefore the classroom teacher will change tactics, for example, giving an assignment instead of a test or vice versa. The bottom line is to find a way to make an exceptional student find success and move forward academically.

Psycho educational assessment is one way to identify students with exceptionalities. In most cases of identification, the classroom teacher will be the first person to recognize signs of a student's exceptionality or exceptionalities. In the province of Ontario, the Identification, Placement and Review Committee (IPRC) is a means of properly identifying students with exceptionalities. This committee works together to decide whether to identify a student as exceptional and, if so, what is the appropriate academic placement should be. This process has allowed teachers to maximize students learning potential as they progress from one tear to the next. Of equal importance, the IPRC is integral to the development of a student's Individualized Education Plan (IEP). Thus, the

IPRC works to properly identify students with exceptionalities and to address the unique needs of each students. There are a number of steps the committee must perform when identifying students with exceptionalities. They start off by taking into consideration an educational assessment of the student; then obtain and consider a health or psychological assessment. If the student is 16 years or older, the IPRC "shall consider any information about the pupil submitted by the parent and pupil," (Brown, 2004, 81). This committee must have three or more people on it, and one of them must be a principal who is employed by the school board; a supervisory officer employed by the school board; and the schools psycho-ed consultant.

THE IMPORTANCE OF ASSESSMENT

Students with mild forms of exceptionalities are now routinely integrated with their peers in the same class, making the classroom teacher responsible for the identified student. The most important role that classroom teachers need to play is identifying students during normal classroom assessments, through tests and assignments. When discrepancies arise as soon as students are not meeting curriculum expectations, it is up to the classroom teacher to contact the parents or guardian of the student. At the same time the teacher will consult with either the school guidance counsellor or directly with the special education teacher. Then he or she should complete necessary referral forms. Once students are identified, they may become eligible for special education services.

When students are identified they go through a series of formal tests. For many years, psychologists within each individual school board have been assessing student with exceptionalities. Before the testing can happen, the classroom teacher, parent, principal and school psychologist meets to discuss the students' needs. Once their meeting has concluded if they have agreed to go a complete academic evaluation on them, then this is done using diagnostic testing as well as an array of psychometric techniques. These tests will evaluate a student's cognitive-intellectual personality as well as their academic functioning. Once all the appropriate assessments are complete, then the psychologists will write up a complete review indicating the student's academic needs. The next step is to reconvene a meeting with the same staff that was present at the earlier IPRC meeting. The psychologist will now address his or her findings and thoroughly explain the results of the testing. At this point, the psychologist will clearly identify the student's strengths and provide many examples; they will also describe the students' needs in their report. This is the most important aspect as it clearly outlines all of the areas of concern, and they are ready for the next step, which is implementation of the IEP.

This implementation of a student's IEP takes place in the classroom. I believe that this is a very important step for classroom teachers to consider carefully. The teacher is now able to review the student's IEP, and come to a complete understanding of their strengths and weaknesses. With help from the psychologist, classroom teachers will map out strategies to benefit the student. As a result, the teacher must now identify the classroom instruction needs and how they are to be modified, in order to ensure success for the student. The teacher's responsibility now is to set short and long term learning targets, and specify the criteria and evaluation procedures that will be used to monitor the academic progress, towards meeting the targets set up. The teacher will set these targets, taking into account the identified strengths, weaknesses and needs in the IEP. It is up to the teacher to set up appropriate tests to use in the classroom that will provide the necessary results to determine whether or not the student is making acceptable progress towards meeting learning targets, again as specified in the IEP. Finally, teachers are responsible for ensuring that the student will participate in regular classroom activities as much as possible.

Based on the students needs some adaptations in terms of testing may also need to be put in place. Some students with exceptionalities will require specific testing accommodations, such as a separate room to write a test in, or a quite room with fewer distractions. As long as a teacher can monitor the testing, and provide students with ample opportunity to complete the test, hopefully they will achieve better results.

When it comes to assisting students with exceptionalities, it is important for special education teachers to know the difference between accommodations and modifications, as these two terms greatly differ from one another. While analyzing students IEPs teachers need to become aware of different aspects of the curriculum that needs to be modified, and then implement the accommodations to help the student with their courses. Accommodations are supports or services that are not provided to the general student population, however they are required by individual students with special needs to help them achieve learning expectations and demonstrate learning. Whereas modifications are changes in the curriculum to help the student academically succeed.

Teaching students with exceptionalities can be a tricky job. It is important to provide supports that are suitable to their needs. When providing students with accommodations, these can range from technological equipment, support staff, and informal supports. Accommodations are different from modifications because they are more of a support service that the student will use to reach the goals of the curriculum. Accommodations are changing how the student learns. For example, providing the students with a computer or note taker to help them with their writing is an example of an accommodation that some students may need. During my practical teaching experiences I have had to incorporate accommodations into my lesson plans as I had a student with a learning disability (LD) in one of my classes. One of the most common accommodations that students with LD needs is breaking up work and giving students extra time to complete their work. Student with LD may feel overwhelmed and tend to work on assignments better when given in small increments. When working with students who have exceptionalities it is important to know that no single method always works. Teachers need to individualize their efforts when accommodating students, as no student is the same.

As each academic year progresses and short term and long term goals are being met, classroom teachers must continually refer to the students` IEP to make appropriate lesson plan accommodations and modifications. Throughout the year, special education teachers will meet with the students' parents or guardian and discuss their child's progress. This is where any accommodations and modifications will be improved or new ones will be implemented. Consultations with the psych-ed personnel will then be conducted for continual support, and further examination of annual goals will take place. These goals should be measurable, positive, student-oriented and relevant, in order for the student to be successful. Finally, at the end of the year, a concluding IPRC meeting will be conducted, where the committee will look at what worked well for the student, and what needs to be improved, and then begin to map out strategies for the up coming academic year.

My future classroom

As a teacher I foresee my classroom as a place where students are welcome from all walks of life. Whether I am a regular classroom teacher, a special education teacher, chaplain or guidance counsellor, I want students to feel comfortable in my presence. It's important for teachers to recognize that students are coming to us with all kinds of ideas, problems, etc. I believe that it is the teacher's moral responsibility to create a positive learning environment for students. I am a Catholic educator and I plan and hope to teach within a Catholic school system. Although many feel that the Catholic system is unfair and we as Catholics should not be given priority over other religions, I sympathize with other faiths. However, working in a Catholic school gives me a sense of faith and comfort. Whether you are teaching religion, science, and geography etc., Catholic teachers have the great responsibility on intertwining Catholic values into their daily lesson plans.

On the York Catholic District School Board's website, they have an interesting quote that I would like to share. It goes like this:

"We are a Catholic Learning Community of collaborative partners, called to serve one another by being committed to and accountable for quality learning by all with Jesus as our inspiration."

To have an education board that is inspired by Jesus and His teachings is awesome for us Catholics. I also believe that it is important for all teachers to try and look for the face of Jesus in all of our co-workers and students. I know and understand that this can be an impossible task, and I am first to admit that there have been times where I have failed to look for the face of Jesus in others, but I believe that if we begin to do this, especially with those who have disabilities, we will begin to see a change in how we treat one another.

I also believe that it is important to make society better aware of people with exceptionalities. This can be done within schools, the workplace and the community. The more people see others with exceptionalities in positions of responsibility, the more they will become more comfortable in their presence. I have often seen people look at me and wonder why I walk or talk differently. It hurts to see people whispering behind my back, and trust me I see it. I would much rather people approach me and ask me about my disability. I am more then happy to talk to people about my challenges and explain to them why I am different from others. Whenever I am out in the community people ask my parents or whoever I am with, "what it wrong with him?" or "why does he speak (or walk) funny?" Then I pipe up and say, "Well, why don't you ask me?" It is so funny to see people's reaction when I respond. And it is even funnier when they are shocked after finding out I have a college diploma, a university and teaching degree.

We need to try our best to make society more aware and comfortable around people with exceptionalities. This can be done in many ways; the most effective way is through educational workshops or seminars. There has always been talk about creating a barrier-free society. Well, I also believe that this needs to include everything; number one priority should be creating a barrier-free work environment.

We now live in a society where disability is a norm, or should be. We have come so far in integrating people with exceptionalities in to the classroom, workplace and in our communities. Thanks to organizations such as Participation House, Ontario Federation for Cerebral Palsy, L'Arche, Christian Blind Mission and many others, they have helped and continue to help increase the quality of life for individuals living with physical and cognitive exceptionalities. We see people with all kinds of exceptionalities within our communities, but do we really understand what they have to deal with on a daily bases. Depending of an individual's age, severity of their disability, cognitive abilities as well as many other factors, simple daily tasks can be challenging to perform. I know for myself, it is hard for me to tie a simple shoelace or dental floss my teeth, but can you imagine those who can not walk or communicate with others. We can all learn from individuals with exceptionalities, and this is why I believe that it is important for me to obtain a teaching position.

When students with and without exceptionalities see professionals who have disabilities working in prestige professions, this can encourage them to work hard for themselves and succeed as well. There is nothing greater in life then achieving your dreams and doing what you do best. I am reminded by the great Dr. Seuss who said in his book, *Oh the Places You'll Go!* "And will you succeed? Yes! You will, indeed! (98 and ¾ percent guaranteed.) Kid, you'll move mountains!" No matter what paths we take in life, I believe that with hard work and dedication we will all be successful.

My late Uncle Jimmy once said to me at my high school graduation party, "successful people have a certain look and way about them, Pete; you have that way and look." His words along with Dr. Seuss' have always been apart of who I am and have helped to encourage me to continue working hard. I believe that with hard work and perseverance, I will eventually land a full time teaching position.

With all that I have learned along with my practical teaching experience and volunteering in schools, there is no doubt that the classroom is a place where I want to be. I have tried working in offices at a 9 to 5 job, and it is not for me. For me teaching is like breathing, I need to work as a teacher in order to fulfill my lifelong dream and live a happy and full life. Put me in the classroom and I am in my element. The classroom is a place where I can grow as a teacher and work with students year after year to help them become the next physicist, person who cures cancer or any dream that they may have. To have the opportunity to educate today's youth for tomorrows future is an awesome responsibility, and I am more then capable and ready to embark on this journey.

WHAT I AM DOING TO TRY AND IMPROVE MY OVERALL PHYSICAL ABILITIES!

I realize that I have physical challenges in life and my speech is not clear, however, through my volunteering and daily interactions with staff and students, I am really trying my best. I need to work on my clarity and pronunciation of words; this is really difficult for me to do. So many times I have broken down and cried over frustration. I constantly ask God why He made me the way I am. Sometime I understand, but most of the time I have a hard time.

I question, did God make a mistake when He created me? Did he not spend as much time on me as he did on others? But then I realize that God is perfect and He doesn't make any mistakes. I try each and every day to wake up and put on a smile, but so many times I just brake down and cry. Yes, I am in my late twenties and I cry. Lately I have been crying a lot. I try and keep my emotions hidden, and on the most part, I do a pretty good job. However, when I cry, I let it out, sometimes with a friend or family member, but mostly on my own. Am I depressed? I wouldn't say that's the case. I have refused to see a therapist, because I know he or she can't remove my disability, or fix my speech. If I could have one of these wishes granted to me, I would rather have a physical disability for the rest of my life, and have perfect speech. I have talked to my family doctor about my speech and the way I walk, and all I need to do is to keep practicing and working on my speech and physical exercises.

For about a year I was having trouble with both of my ankles. They were really hurting, to the point where I couldn't walk. My family doctor sent me to an orthopedic surgeon, and I told him about my ankle pains. The first visit it was mostly my right ankle that was bothering so I had the cortisone shot in my one ankle. After a while it started feeling a lot better. My ankle wasn't tightening and locking up, it felt great. Then a few months later my left ankle started hurting. Instead of going back to my family doctor, I contacted Dr. Haider again. Fortunately, I didn't need another referral, I was immediately scheduled to go in for another cortisone shot, and so far, *knock on wood*, the pain in both ankles have subsided. I'm hoping it won't come back in the near future. I do have some pain now and then, but not as much as I used to. Now all I need to fix is my speech and ego.

Living with a disability is very hard. Although my case of CP is mild, I do face challenges each and everyday of my life. There is so much that I want to do in life and places I want to see, but often my disability limits me from doing many activities. I would love to teach overseas. I have been offered three positions as a teacher in Australia, China and London, England. I applied just for fun and did receive a few calls. The only reason why I didn't take any of the offers was because I wasn't sure how to arrange transportation to work and around town. I also need assistance from time to time with daily activities, like cutting up meat, cooking, ironing, and a few others. Although teaching overseas would be a rich experience for me; and I encourage all teachers to try this at least once in their career, this is one experience that would be challenging for me to do. Rarely do I ever say that something is impossible for me to do or overcome, because I know that with God all things are possible. However, I do have to realize that I am an individual with a disability, and I do have limitations that I need to face and learn to accept. This is hard for me to do at many times in my life.

WHAT TEACHERS NEED TO KNOW!

I want to end my story with sharing what I believe that teachers need to know. Teaching is a profession that calls professionals to work in collaboration with their colleagues in order to improve the delivery of the curriculum to our students. The standards of practice for the teaching profession are important for teachers to take into consideration as they are meant to inspire a shared vision for all teachers and identify the values, knowledge and skills that are distinctive. The standards are also there to help guide professional judgement and daily actions. Lastly, they promote a common language that fosters an understanding of what it means to be a valuable member of the teaching profession.

Being committed to teaching and students is extremely imperative for all educators to do. It is crucial for teachers to care for students equitably and with respect, while being sensitive to the factors that influences their learning. I believe that it is important for teachers to show that they are interested in the learning process of students, and we need to treat students like important individuals who are valuable contributors to our Canadian society. By being committed to our students and their learning, will help them develop their skills and strive for excellence as they continue on their education paths.

The standards of practice for the teaching profession are important for teachers to take into consideration as they are meant to inspire a shared vision for all teachers and identify the values, knowledge and skills that are distinctive. The standards are also there to help guide professional judgement and daily actions. Lastly, they promote a common language that fosters an understanding of what it means to be a valuable member of the teaching profession.

In order to effectively teach any academic or applied level subjects, teachers must recognize the importance of professional knowledge. It is vital for teachers to stay current in this profession and constantly reflect on their students' development, learning theory, pedagogy, curriculum, ethics, and education research. Teachers also need to be in touch with educational polices and legislation in order to improve professional judgement throughout their profession. One way teachers can advance their professional knowledge is through constantly educating themselves. This can be done by taking additional qualification courses, attending professional workshops/seminars, and keeping themselves up to date with knowledge of educational practices and issues within their community. With their professional knowledge teachers can effectively apply it to their practice and promote student learning.

As teachers it is also important to remember that we are all leaders within our school communities. It is imperative that we work together with our colleagues to make our schools a collaborative, safe and supportive learning community for all members. In order to facilitate student success teachers must recognize their shared responsibilities as well as their leadership roles that will help them be a part of their student's achievement. Since we are called to be professionals, we must maintain and uphold the principles of ethical standards when working within our learning communities as we are constantly role models for our students. Teachers need to realize that teaching is a profession that involves ongoing learning on their part. It is important for teachers to frequently educate themselves in order to effectively teach their students and keep up with the changes in education to help their students succeed. When teachers exercise these five standards it allows them to become actively involved in practicing and improving their teaching methods and strategies. Teaching is an important profession that should be entered into with deep dedication and commitment. When teachers absolutely love what they do, this encourages them to improve their skills and become better teachers to educate and improve the future of their students.

With their professional knowledge teachers can effectively apply it to their practice and promote student learning. In order to perfect their practice, teachers need to use appropriate pedagogy, assessment and evaluation strategies, as well as resources, technology and tactics that will effectively help them plan, respond to the needs of their students and enhance the learning environment.

As teachers it is also important to remember that we are all leaders within our school communities. It is imperative that we work together with our colleagues to make our schools a collaborative, safe and supportive learning community for all members. In order to facilitate student success teachers must recognize their shared responsibilities as well as their leadership roles that will help them be a part of their student's achievement. Since we are called to be professionals, we must maintain and uphold the principles of ethical standards when working within our learning communities as we are constantly role models for our students.

Lastly, teachers need to realize that teaching is a profession that involves ongoing learning on their part. It is important for teachers to frequently educate themselves in order to effectively teach their students and keep up with the changes in education to help their students succeed. When teachers exercise these five standards it allows them to become actively involved in practicing and improving their teaching methods and strategies. Teaching is an important profession that should be entered into with deep dedication and commitment. When teachers absolutely love what they do, this encourages them to improve their skills and become better teachers to educate and improve the future of their students.

CO-OPERATIVE LEARNING

Working with students with exceptionalities is an awesome experience. As a qualified teacher I strongly believe that students with exceptionalities need to be integrated in the schools as much as possible. One way that I find successful is through cooperative learning. When students with exceptionalities are placed in co-operative learning environments with non-disabled peers, this requires the students to not only learn new skills and better their existing skills, this also allows them to co-operate with their peers. It furthermore permits them to get a sense of satisfaction from improving their overall academic abilities. Right now many students with exceptionalities are participating in a modified program that allows them to partake in their school environment but at the same time, differs from the regular program. In many cases, special education teachers need to be very careful on how much support a student needs. Too much support can affect student's ability to motivate themselves. As teachers we need to see what students can do for themselves, and then implement special services when needed. Integration may be the key to personal growth and success for students with mild exceptionalities. Exploring the benefits of cooperative learning will help educators create a learning environment that is inviting to all students especially those identified with exceptionalities. As a prospective teacher, I strongly believe that the socialization process of students should be closely linked to the educational process, as this is important for teenagers when maturing into an adult and making decision with respect to others.

The definition of co-operative learning is the process of acquiring knowledge in a socially packed environment by small groups learning together and taking advantage of each other's expertise to achieve a common goal (Faryadi 2007, 2). Therefore, the purpose of co-operative learning is to promote the inclusion among students with exceptionalities in the general education classroom. Co-operative learning

"is categorized by classroom techniques that involve students in group learning activities, in which recognition and reinforcement are based on groups, rather than individual performance," (Smith et al., 2006, 348).

When teachers encourage co-operative learning in their classrooms, this allows non-disabled students to work with students who have exceptionalities, and together they achieve group goals and student success for all. There are many successful strategies that teachers can implement when promoting co-operative learning. "These include peer tutoring, group projects, the jigsaw technique, and student-team achievement division," (Smith et al., 2006, 348).

One important concept for co-operative learning is known as student-team achievement division (STAD). This involves assigning students to groups that meet to discuss and review teacher-generated lessons. The STAD technique employs three main concepts, which include: team rewards, individual accountability, and equal opportunities for success. It is important to promote individual accountability as it essential for all to learn the content in order for their team to be academically successful. "Co-operative learning strategies offer much promise as inclusive practices," (Smith et al., 2006, 349). By implementing co-operative learning, this can be successful for low, average, as well as high achievers as it promotes academic success and social skill that help enhance their independence. Co-operative leaning can also boost the social adjustment of students with exceptionalities and assist them in creating support networks. Although co-operative learning is not suitable for all types of exceptionalities, it is a beneficial technique for students with physical exceptionalities as well as students with mild forms of learning exceptionalities.

In my teaching experiences, one important component to co-operative learning is the peer tutoring approach. This is a relatively easy-to-manage system that teachers can execute in their classroom. Teachers can assign high-achievers to work one-on-one with students with exceptionalities, and credit them based on their cooperation and tutoring efforts. This technique "can benefit both the student being tutored and the tutor," (Smith et al., 2006, 348). When working with peers it is important to encourage students with exceptionalities to be in the center of learning. When students work alongside their peers this improves their critical thinking and intellectual skills. Co-operative learning is very promising; the promise is to encourage students to become active learners and work constructively with their peers. Many teachers "feel that co-operative learning is an effective strategy to decrease off-task behaviour and promotes positive skills, so [they] would recommend using this as an intervention," (Pate-Clevenger et al., 2008, 66). This is one of the many teaching techniques that I hope to use in my future classroom.

Ever since I have struggled to find a job, it has been my goal to make myself physically better and improve the quality of my life. Improving my physical abilities is important to me, because I need to prove to people that there is more to me then my disability. Shortly after graduation my family doctor sent me to a neurologist to assess my speech and walking. Like other specialist there was nothing that she could really recommend, other then getting back into physiotherapy and speech therapy. After the assessment the neurologist sent me to West Park Healthcare Center where they have a team of doctors and therapist helping adults with exceptionalities improve their quality of life. Since 1904 this healthcare center has been helping people manage difficult health challenges. This center first began as a sanitarium for patients with tuberculoses, and later expanded their services to helping those with lung disease, diabetes, stroke, amputation and musculoskeletal issues.

I would recommend this health care facility to anyone living with a physical disability, or any disability for that matter. Living with CP as an adult has been very challenging for me. Not only has it been had to find a job, I am finding it even more challenging to prove to prospective employers that I have so much to offer to many organizations. My exceptionality is just physical, yet so many people get the wrong impression of me, and think I have learning challenges as well. Everyday I try my best to improve my walking and speech. I have been doing both speech and physical therapy at West Park, and have received a number of botox treatments in my right arm and leg to help reduce the tightness which is caused from spasticity.

The biggest challenge I am dealing with is proving to people that there is more to who I am then my physical challenges. Yes, CP is a neurological disorder, however since there are many types of disabilities, I am considered to be high functioning. It might take me longer to get from point A to point B, but there is nothing wrong with my intellectual abilities.

We need to somehow make society more accepting and tolerant to individuals with physical exceptionalities. If more employers' hirer educated and qualified people with exceptionalities, then I believe that these individuals will begin to receive more respect from society at large. Instead of looking at a person with an exceptionality and wondering why they are different, I want to encourage people to approach more individuals, like myself and find out our story. No one who sees me for the first time would ever imagine that I have a college diploma and two university degrees under my belt. Individuals who just have physical challenges can offer so much to society if they are given the chance to prove themselves.

This journey of mine has inspired me to write my story and share it with others. I want people to know that no matter what challenges we face in life, it is important to keep a strong faith in God and continue trying out best. My parents, family members, and close friends keep telling me to stay strong and never give up; they promise me that something will come up. Although this is tough to do and trust me I have had my moments were I have vented my frustration to my family and friends. However, this has only taught me that venting and showing anger gets you no where in life. So I have decided to continue volunteering in schools, participate as a sponsor for the RCIA committee through my Church, and wait until God tells me that I am ready to work. I know that one day I will obtain a teaching position and I will be the best teacher and continue to inspire my students and colleagues. When it comes to the end of the day, the fact is that I have worked so hard and have accomplished so much, and all I can say is that I belong in the classroom. If I can get this far in life, then so can you. All I need to do is find a principal who will look past my disability and see my inner teacher spirit. If I am given an opportunity to prove to the world that I can in fact maintain a teaching career, I know that I will succeed, just like I have many times over in the past.

Thank you all for reading my story!!! God Bless.

REFERENCES

Brown, Anthony F. *Legal Handbook for Educators.* Thomson Canada Limited, 2004. Print.

Coloroso, Barbara. *Parenting With Wit And Wisdom.* Penguin Group Canada, 2003. Print.

Pate-Clevenger, Rebecca, and Dusing, Jennifer, et al. (2008). Improving Off-Task Behaviour of Elementary and High School Students Through the use of Co-operative Learning. Retrieved Jan. 23, 2011 from http://www.ericdigests.org/.

Smith, Tom E.C. et al. *Teaching Students with Special Needs in Inclusive Settings.* Toronto, Ontario: Pearson Education Canada Inc., 2006. Print.

Ontario College of Teachers. *The Ethical Standards for the Teaching Profession*. 2006.

Ontario Ministry of Education. (2001). Special Education: A Guide for Educators. http://www.edu.gov.on.ca/eng/general/elemsec/speced/guide.html.

ABOUT THE AUTHOR

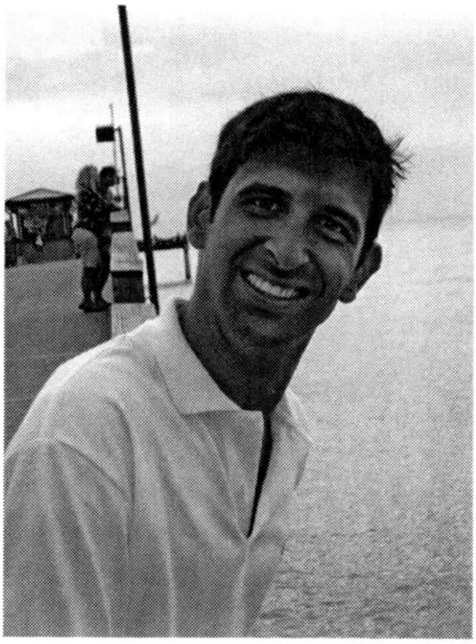

Peter Daniel Mitskinis is a qualified teacher in Ontario, who has Cerebral Palsy. Peter first started his academic journey with the hopes of becoming a Journalist. After receiving his Ontario College Diploma, he realized that this was not the career path for him. He then fell in love with teaching through his volunteer experiences in local elementary and high schools within their special education departments.

With the inspiration of becoming a special education teacher, school chaplain and guidance counsellor, Peter received his Bachelor of Arts degree as well as his Bachelor of Professional

Studies in Education degree. With qualifications in Religious Studies, Geography, Special Education as well as Guidance and Career Education, Peter strives to obtain a teaching position where he can work with youth of all ages, and continue to inspire others to pursue their own dreams in life.

Despite what challenges Peter has been faced with, his story is a living proof of how successful anybody can be no matter what limitations one might be faced with. His advice to all who are fortunate enough to read his book is, if you have a goal in mind and want to pursue a career that you are passionate about, do not let anyone or anything stop you from pursuing your dreams. Peter wants to encourage individuals both with and without exceptionalities to continue striving for success, and whenever a roadblock may present itself, always keep a strong faith in God, because with God anything is possible. He is a living proof of that!

To learn more about Peter or even contact him, please continue to follow his journey by visiting his blog: www.ibelongintheclassroom.com.

Office de la propriété intellectuelle du Canada

Un organisme d'Industrie Canada

Canadian Intellectual Property Office

An Agency of Industry Canada

Certificate of Registration of

Copyright

Certificat d'enregistrement du

Droit d'auteur

This Certificate of Registration is issued pursuant to sections 49 and 53 of the Copyright Act. The copyright in the work described below was registered on the date of registration as follows:

Ce certificat d'enregistrement est émis conformément aux articles 49 et 53 de la Loi sur le droit d'auteur. Le droit d'auteur sur l'oeuvre décrite ci-dessous, a été enregistré à la date d'enregistrement comme suit :

Date of Registration - Date d'enregistrement : **July 10, 2012**

Registration No. - Numéro d'enregistrement : **1096992**

First Publication - Première publication : **Unpublished**

Title - Titre : **I Belong in the Classroom**

Category - Catégorie : **Literary**

Owner(s) - Titulaire(s) :
Peter Mitskinis
106 Stephensbrook Circle
Stouffville, Ontario
Canada, L4A 0G5

Author(s) - Auteur(s) : **Peter Mitskinis**

Peter Mitskinis

Date of Issuance of Certificate - Date d'émission du certificat : **July 10, 2012**

Registrar of Copyright / Copyright office — Registraire des droits d'auteur / Bureau du droit d'auteur

Canada

CIPO 0C200 (09-11)

OPIC CIPO

CPSIA information can be obtained at www.ICGtesting.com
Printed in the USA
BVOW010614210912

301033BV00001B/3/P